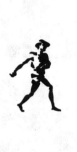

THE

SOUTHAMPTON
DIET

Stuart Berger, M.D.

WITH

MARCIA COHEN

SIMON AND SCHUSTER • NEW YORK

COPYRIGHT © 1982 BY STUART BERGER, M.D.
ALL RIGHTS RESERVED
INCLUDING THE RIGHT OF REPRODUCTION
IN WHOLE OR IN PART IN ANY FORM
PUBLISHED BY SIMON AND SCHUSTER
A DIVISION OF GULF & WESTERN CORPORATION
SIMON & SCHUSTER BUILDING
ROCKEFELLER CENTER
1230 AVENUE OF THE AMERICAS
NEW YORK, NEW YORK 10020
SIMON AND SCHUSTER AND COLOPHON ARE TRADEMARKS OF SIMON
& SCHUSTER
DESIGNED BY EVE METZ
MANUFACTURED IN THE UNITED STATES OF AMERICA

LIBRARY OF CONGRESS CATALOGING IN PUBLICATION DATA

BERGER, STUART.
　　THE SOUTHAMPTON DIET.

　　　INCLUDES INDEX.
　　　1. REDUCING DIETS.　2. REDUCING DIETS—RECIPES.
3. REDUCING DIETS—MENUS.　I. COHEN, MARCIA.　II. TITLE.
RM222.2.B4524　　　613.2'5　　　82-5502
ISBN 0-671-44525-1　　　　　　AACR2

We are most grateful to Kathy Colligan for her nutritional expertise, to Jenni Stone for her painstaking work on the recipes, to Kim Honig for her research, development and editing of the recipes, to Mark Fuerst for his aid in research, to Juanita Butler for her recipe testing and to Louise Fisher for manuscript preparation.

We are equally indebted to the excellent team assembled by Simon and Schuster: Michael Korda, John Herman, Dan Green, Julia Knickerbocker, Wendy Sherman, Rebecca Head, Judy Lee and Al Reuben.

And . . . for their enduring support we would like to thank our families: Rachel, Otto, Anna, Belle, Larry, Betsy and Jesse, as well as special friends Dick Kaplan, Irving Lazar, Susan Kasen, Robert Walker, Phyllis Levy, Gordon Weaver and Judy Kamen.

Many others—too numerous to mention here—have been helpful and encouraging and our gratitude extends to them as well.

This book is dedicated to people
who pursue their goals
through good health

CONTENTS

1 • I KNOW WHAT IT'S LIKE TO BE FAT—THE BIRTH OF THE
     SOUTHAMPTON DIET   11
2 • WHY THE SOUTHAMPTON DIET WORKS—WHERE OTHERS
     HAVE FAILED   30
3 • THE FAT SHIELD—YOUR WORST ENEMY   46
4 • THE BIOCHEMICAL MIRACLE—MOOD AND FOOD   61
5 • HAPPY FOODS, SAD FOODS   70
6 • SEX AND YOUR WEIGHT   77
7 • HOW TO STAY ON THE SOUTHAMPTON DIET   90
8 • THE SOUTHAMPTON DIET CONTRACT   103

THE DIETS   107
THE SOUTHAMPTON DIET MENU, 109
THE SOUTHAMPTON RESTAURANT AND
     VACATION MENU, 129

THE ETHNIC DIETS   139
FRENCH AND NOUVELLE CUISINE MENU, 143
ITALIAN MENU, 152
JAPANESE MENU, 161
CHINESE MENU, 171
GREEK MENU, 181
MEXICAN MENU, 189
JEWISH MENU, 198

9

CONTENTS

THE SOUTHAMPTON MAINTENANCE DIET, 206
QUESTIONS AND ANSWERS, 224

THE RECIPES   235
THE SOUTHAMPTON DIET RECIPES, 237
FRENCH AND NOUVELLE CUISINE RECIPES, 244
ITALIAN RECIPES, 261
JAPANESE RECIPES, 276
CHINESE RECIPES, 290
GREEK RECIPES, 300
MEXICAN RECIPES, 315
JEWISH RECIPES, 326
THE SOUTHAMPTON MAINTENANCE DIET
          RECIPES, 338

APPENDIX   341

INDEX   349

1

I KNOW WHAT IT'S LIKE TO BE FAT—THE BIRTH OF THE SOUTHAMPTON DIET

YOU BOUGHT THIS BOOK because you want to be thin.

It would be foolish to deny that in today's world, thin people are beautiful people. They are also, not incidentally, healthier and happier people

In past eras—when Peter Paul Rubens painted his fleshy nudes, for instance—the high premium we place on slender, supple good looks simply didn't exist. In short, fat was fine in the seventeenth century.

It is always possible, of course, that our standards will change again someday, and that the superabundant body will charm us all once more. I seriously doubt that this will happen, however. All the evidence medical science has accumulated thus far points to obesity as a major health hazard. Statistics on the overweight portion of our population show an excess mortality rate of up to thirty percent,

11

resulting from diseases of the heart and blood vessels, diabetes, cerebral hemorrhage, cancer, accidents and suicide.

The fact that even the suicide rate is high among overweight people supports the major premise of this book.

I firmly believe that, in the modern world, we would be hard put to find a factor more damaging to an individual's self-esteem and life goals than the demeaning and energy-depleting baggage of overweight. Today, a slender body is almost always equated with power, success and happiness. We even tend to distrust people who are grossly overweight, to regard them as less intelligent and well-disciplined than those who are slim.

That last statement may seem surprisingly harsh, but if you think about it, you will probably admit that it is accurate. In the United States today it would be almost impossible for a fat man to be elected president. Our heroes and heroines are invariably thin.

Because of my own personal experience with obesity—which you will read about later in this chapter—I take the problem of overweight, even if it is only a few pounds, very seriously. Not every doctor does. *I* do.

"Thinness" is a perfectly rational, logical goal in our twentieth-century world, not only because medical science has shown us the damaging physical effects of overweight but also because of what we see with our own eyes every day. To be thin, in most cases, is to be happy and energetic, full of hope and a buoyant joy in being alive.

Nowhere is the importance of this goal, this slender body, more evident than in Southampton, Long Island, the location of one of my offices.

Southampton, as many of you probably know, is one section of the famous and luxurious Hamptons, far out on the eastern tip of Long Island. This is the chic "in" resort area for trendy and successful people in New York City, the background for many of the brilliant photographs you see in fashion magazines and the setting for some of the most magnificent homes in the world. Rambling estates belonging to wealthy and aristocratic families like the Du Ponts and the Fords are dotted along the thirty-mile coastline, their emerald-green lawns and prize-winning gardens rimmed with high, sculptured hedges and hundreds of feet of fragrant, honeysuckle-laden fences.

The towns in the Hamptons are showplaces for the most imaginative artists and designers in the New York area; the small shops are filled with marvels of the antique and the avant-garde. The pale clear light at this far point on the island is so compelling that artists such as Jackson Pollock and Georgia O'Keeffe painted some of their greatest works here.

Just as the boutiques and art galleries of the Hamptons cater to the most sophisticated artistic eye, so do the restaurants attend to the most cultivated taste. Their menus range from the fashionable nouvelle cuisine to hearty steak and lobster meals, and there is an array of ethnic bistros that cater to the vast range of Manhattan's multinational population. Food critics Craig Claiborne, Pierre Franey and James Beard must be satisfied in these splendid restaurants, just as residents such as Ralph Lauren and Lauren Bacall must be pleased in the elegant shops.

In short, the Hamptons are a weekend and summer playground for some of the most powerful figures in the arts— famous names and faces from television, film and publishing. Dina Merrill summers here, as do Truman Capote, Eli Wallach and Anne Jackson, Diana Ross, Mick Jagger, Kurt Vonnegut, Andy Warhol, William Paley, George Plimpton, Richard Avedon, Bob Fosse—and on and on. Jacqueline Kennedy Onassis and Lee Radziwill spent their early summers here, at the Maidstone Country Club in East Hampton.

But the Hamptons are not exclusively inhabited by the

already rich and famous. Young people in all sorts of highly competitive fields—actors and actresses, up-and-coming models and writers, lawyers and physicians and stockbrokers—also spend many happy hours on the Hamptons' wide, white, sunny beaches.

One can hardly avoid noticing the importance of slender, healthy bodies to these beautiful people in Southampton. On the beach, of course, they wear very little clothing; off the beach they are extremely conscious of how they look in the fashionable clothes they do wear. The connection between physical appearance and success in a high-powered world is obvious.

In Southampton, thin is the name of the game, and the game is that of living a richly creative and happy life. To be overweight is to be deprived of the social, psychological and often even financial rewards of this dazzling community.

But how do these attractive people achieve and maintain this enviable state? How do the Beautiful People stay beautiful?

Few alert and knowledgeable people in Southampton or anywhere else will—or should—tolerate diets that deprive them of energy, good health or high spirits . . . or even diets that can't be maintained over a long period of time. In Southampton, dieters demand a program of weight loss that is *always* both successful and healthy.

The program I have devised for my patients is therefore one that has been molded on my own experience of losing 210 pounds and keeping that weight off.

In a sense, I myself was "born-again thin." Because I was able to lose the weight, my life changed radically.

Need I say "for the better"? Of course not.

I am a happy man today, and this book is written to teach you—as I have taught my patients—how to achieve that same happiness for yourself. Since thin is the name of the game, you will play that game. You will never again sit on the sidelines (as I once did) watching the other players carry off the spoils of success—friends, financial rewards or the applause of one's peers.

Of course we are all born with handicaps of one sort or another that limit our success in certain fields. (We can't be ballet dancers if we are born with flat feet.) Fat is also a handicap. Fat also limits our success.

But no one is born fat! At some point or points in our lives, we learned to inflict this cruel punishment on ourselves.

Unlike ballet dancing, being thin is not a goal any one of us is unequipped to achieve. Not everyone can dance with the New York City Ballet, but everyone *can* reach a body weight that will provide a successful, happy life.

But attaining—and maintaining—that happy state is not a simple task—no matter what the current diet "guru" may be proclaiming to the world at large. We all need help along this difficult road.

With this book, I intend to provide you with all the help you need. As a physician, psychiatrist and dieter myself, I will be your guide and, I hope, your friend.

I have discovered over many years of study that there are definite biochemical, nutritional and psychological factors involved in weight loss and that these factors strongly affect the dieting process.

An understanding of these three elements in dieting is what changed my life, and it will do the same thing for you. You will, as I did, learn to stop punishing yourself into extra pounds, and nurture yourself into a happy, healthy weight loss instead.

Because I once weighed 420 pounds (which even at six feet six-and-a-half inches tall is obese) and because I successfully shed that weight, I have a deep and thorough understanding of the problems associated with dieting. I understand these problems—not only for those who must lose a large amount of weight but for those who only want to lose a few pounds. For some people—and I am one of them—four to ten added pounds can signal a good deal of emotional and physical discomfort, not the least of which is adding those pounds year after year until they are no longer just a few.

As a physician, I have a lifelong commitment to maintaining the highest possible level of physical health in my patients. As a psychiatrist, I am concerned with mental health. It is this combination—the personal, medical and psychiatric—that led to the creation of *The Southampton Diet*.

The Southampton Diet program is not exclusively a plan for those who must lose weight to the extent that I did. After all, when I lost 210 pounds, I lost almost as much as two average women weigh. I lost half my own weight and found myself with an entirely new image. Instead of a six-feet six-and-a-half-inch elephant, I am now often taken for a professional basketball player.

Still, the factors that led to my enormous weight loss apply as well to those who want to lose much less. They should be taken seriously by any dieter or any physician who is prescribing a weight-loss program.

My own history may be helpful to you not only because it reveals beyond any doubt the reasons for my passionate interest in the subject of weight loss, but because it reflects so many weight problems taken to the extreme.

I grew up in Brooklyn, New York, in a small apartment above a candy store. The candy store itself was, of course, an inducement to weight gain. Milkshakes, ice cream, chocolate syrup were always available.

But *every* child of *every* candy-store owner in the country doesn't become obese! Obviously, other factors were at work. Most of them influenced the formation of the Southampton Diet program, and perhaps some of them will help you understand the principles behind it.

The candy store my parents owned was not a particularly lucrative one, and they were forced to work seven days a week to support us. This meant that they had no opportunity to make friends, and that I, an only child, was somewhat isolated as well.

When I was five years old and just entering kindergarten, my grandmother (my father's mother) came to live with us, and my progressive weight gain dates from this period.

My grandmother, a stern, somewhat overbearing Viennese woman in her late fifties, was given almost total responsibility for my care and discipline. She was an obsessively neat woman, totally oblivious to the rough-and-tumble lifestyle of the average American child. As a result, she dressed her young charge in European-style clothing —white shirts and jackets—which she insisted must remain immaculately clean. Since I obviously could not keep my clothes clean if I was outside playing in the street, I was required to come directly indoors after school.

Indoors, for me, meant the candy store, where as a child I "hung out"—reading, helping my parents with the customers . . . and helping myself to candy bars.

In this environment I became fairly adept at relating to adults but obtained little or no informal experience with children my own age. The school I attended was far outside the neighborhood. I traveled there by bus and returned home immediately after classes ended. I was permitted outside only to visit the next-door neighbor, a little girl named Celeste, whose parents—an Italian butcher and his wife— entertained me with heaping bowls of spaghetti.

Because of my isolation I was supremely unskilled at negotiating childhood relationships. I was shy and ill at ease with my peers, and that shyness, I realized even then (though I had no notion of what to do about it), was misinterpreted by my classmates as a sense of superiority. This was not a very attractive trait to them.

As I grew older—and heavier—I developed another emotional problem. I became painfully embarrassed by the shabbiness of the candy store. This embarrassment further inhibited any attempts on my part to make friends with young people my own age.

By the time I reached junior high school I was already a very lonely young boy, highly insecure and very much in need of warmth and companionship. Celeste had grown into a popular young woman but I was too withdrawn to attempt anything but the most platonic relationship with her. I hid my real feelings for her behind a sort of dogged loyalty. But my loneliness, like any powerful sense of deprivation that is experienced in adolescence, created strong feelings of frustration and anger. These feelings, in turn, were expressed in self-destructive behavior.

But self-destructive behavior, as we all know, is not uncommon in adolescents. Why, in my case, was it manifested in weight gain? Why not—as happens so often—in drug or alcohol abuse?

The answer lies partly in the fact that the subject of weight was an important one in my family. Both my parents were overweight and frustrated by their failure to conquer it. My father was obsessed with dieting and his weight often fluctuated between 200 and 300 pounds every year or two. Then, from time to time, my parents would focus their attention on the ever-present symbol of their frustration—their only son's overweight problem.

Furthermore, one of the great pleasures in this very ethnic home was eating good food. My grandmother was a harsh disciplinarian, but if I behaved well she would cook up a pot of marvelous goulash and noodles. If I was naughty, of course, I was denied that reward.

I hope most of us realize by now that using food for either reward or punishment gives it inordinate importance in a child's mind. My grandmother, however, had no such knowledge of modern psychological theory. Denying me that goulash was a frequent disciplinary measure. If I was late returning home from school, as I was on one particularly memorable occasion (I had remained to help nominate class officers), my goulash was remanded to the refrigerator and I was presented with a plate of despised cold cuts instead.

Thus it happened that this very important domestic issue —food—became a perfect weapon for a young boy in his struggle to grow up. It was a handy and powerful tool of revenge and retribution, a way of "getting back."

This is how it worked.

Since my mother and father, both intelligent people who recognized the potential dangers and emotional distress of overweight, wanted me to be thin, I could "get back" at them by getting fat! I could punish my parents for: one— owning a candy store, and two—incarcerating me in the care of my strict grandmother.

My use of this weapon is well illustrated by what I still think of as the case of the Christmas lasagna.

Each year, on Christmas Eve, an employee in the candy store presented my parents with a huge pan of lasagna. My grandmother always kept that delicious treat in the refrigerator overnight and we all enjoyed it on Christmas Day.

On Christmas Eve of my eleventh year, however, I was particularly furious with my grandmother. She had refused to allow me to go outside all day, in spite of the fact that the first snow of the year had fallen and the streets seemed to me at their brightest and cleanest.

That night, at two o'clock in the morning, I slipped out of bed and headed for the refrigerator. Discovering the lasagna, I systematically consumed every last mouthful. It consisted, I am sure, of at least five pounds of pasta in rich tomato sauce.

The next morning my mother was aghast. The implications of what I had done upset her terribly.

"Stuart, how could you do that?" she asked, her eyes wide with horror. And I answered, with typical insouciance, "I was hungry."

But of course it was more than that. (In fact, I had become somewhat ill from overeating.)

Something else was happening, too, and many of you have sensed it already.

While as an adolescent I was busily, though of course unconsciously, "getting back" at—or punishing—my parents, I was also punishing myself, making myself fatter, more isolated and more miserable every day.

The fact of the matter is that most of us who suffer from weight problems are caught in an awful trap of self-punishment. How we are punished by the outside world and how we learn to punish ourselves is a subject that will be taken up in greater detail in a later chapter. Suffice it to say, at the moment, that this book will teach you how to protect yourself from punishment from others and how to stop punishing yourself here and now.

In my case, as an adolescent I was actually punishing myself while I thought I was giving myself great pleasure, the only pleasure I knew—eating.

In the grip of any negative emotion—anger, for example, or frustration—or when faced with some sort of disappointment to myself, some inability to achieve what I wanted to achieve, I would usually reach for food and devour it. I would, of course, achieve an immediate oral gratification from that act. A sense of quick fulfillment occurred.

Psychiatrists call this "sublimation." I was clearly sublimating my original desire for both companionship and achievement.

20

In short, I *thought* I was making myself happy—or happier than I was. In fact, I was making myself profoundly unhappy and depressed.

It has been many years now since I first became aware of and learned to reverse this self-punishing dynamic. In a later chapter I will show you how to recognize such a characteristic in yourself and how to control it.

In my case, the awareness came about this way:

My unhealthy eating dynamic operated all through my college years. As a result I grew fatter and fatter.

During my summer vacation, between college and medical school, I financed a trip to Paris with a small sum of money I had made from a series of summer jobs.

Paris was a dream come true for me, and the summer was magnificent. One evening I made a date with my friend Debbie, a young woman who attended Bryn Mawr College in the States. We decided to go to the Opéra.

It was a spectacular evening. The boulevards were filled with stunning, well-dressed Parisians, their supple bodies poured into their beautiful, elegantly tailored clothes. Debbie and I joined these marvelous-looking people as we filed into the exquisite Opéra. Debbie looked as lovely as the chic Frenchwomen in the audience, while I, at 420 pounds, plodded along at her side like a circus elephant on parade.

When we reached our places, Debbie sat down. I, meanwhile, slowly lowered my bloated derriere toward my own seat.

But I never reached it.

To my horror, the years of overeating had caught up to me in a moment that could not have been more painful.

I could not fit into the seat.

It was a humiliation I shall never forget. I rushed clumsily out of the Opéra, my eyes brimming with hot, embarrassed tears. I can't recall now how I made my way back to the small pension—only that I spent the night in an agony of self-recrimination.

Not that this was the first time I had experienced difficulty wedging myself into a chair. Obviously, at 420 pounds, embarrassing squeezes had occurred in my life before this moment. They happened every time I traveled by air. Trying to fit into an airplane seat was incredibly difficult and fastening my seat belt an amazing accomplishment.

However, in the past somehow I had always managed to hide my obesity.

Correction! I had always managed to convince my*self* that I was hiding my obesity.

Overweight people will quickly recognize most of these self-delusions:

- I always made sure I was wearing a big, concealing (!) jacket.
- I always tried to sit alone.
- If other passengers were seated near me, I never acknowledged their presence, so as to avoid dealing directly with the intrusion of my extra pounds into their limited space.

But somehow—to my great good fortune—my self-delusion failed me at this moment in the Opéra.

Suddenly what I saw was this:

Paris was beautiful; Debbie was beautiful; and I was excessively ugly.

At that moment, the unhealthy eating dynamic we spoke of earlier no longer worked either. The food that I had in the past convinced myself was a gift of happiness was clearly the opposite. That chewing and swallowing, that immediate oral gratification, was a punishment of the worst kind, bringing me misery, embarrassment and isolation. Something very serious had happened in my mind. *This was a true turning point.* Something had changed.

I embarked on a diet.

Had I never dieted before? Well, of course I had. Up to this point I had tried every new book that was published, every new diet that came along. Each one worked for a week or two. I would often lose ten or twelve pounds, then gain them back, plus another fifteen or twenty pounds.

What was the difference this time? It was, quite simply, the start of a four-point program that I developed gradually over the years. Fad diets were obviously not the answer. I knew that I had to learn more. In the beginning I made many mistakes—most of them typical of any determined person who has not actually learned how to diet.

Immediately after the incident in Paris, I put myself on a 300-calorie-a-day diet—near-starvation. I traveled through Spain for about a week after that, feeling more and more lethargic and depleted; then I flew home. I registered for medical school two days later and headed immediately for the office of a Boston internist for a checkup.

According to the scale, I had lost twenty pounds, but the physician was horrified by my physical condition, my skin tone, incipient flabbiness and other clinical signs of what was, indeed, near-starvation. (Laboratory tests confirmed this unhappy diagnosis.)

The doctor insisted that I change my diet immediately, and I embarked on her prescribed program—a standard nutritional diet. The plan was based on calories and offered many choices within the daily calorie limit. I did continue to lose weight (though at a much slower pace), and the signs of starvation soon faded.

But I was very unhappy. I often felt hungry and had powerful desires to binge. Furthermore, I was carrying a calorie counter everywhere, which was annoying.

Some progress had indeed been made, but not enough. My daily diet was not as balanced as it should have been because I found that I often reached my calorie limit without eating some of the foods needed for proper nutrition. The diet seemed like a department store. There were so many choices that a nutritional balance could easily elude me. And my moodiness was excessive, even for a student under the pressures of the first year of medical school.

I was in Boston, surrounded by the finest scientific and medical minds, yet still having serious difficulties with what I thought should be a simple matter—weight loss. I decided right then to focus my attention on that problem, to learn how the medical and scientific information I was absorbing pertained to what was one of the most important needs in my life.

I began by searching out and reading everything that had been written on the subject of overweight. I found, not surprisingly, that it was the most refractory medical conundrum of our time. It had been attacked with little success by internists, physiologists, psychopharmacologists, nutritionists, neurologists, endocrinologists and even—in the most horrifying manner—by surgeons. In the latter case, a procedure known as "stomach stapling" had been the last in a series of unconscionable surgical interventions.

Amphetamines, often called anorectics or anorexigenics, had been prescribed with little or no clinical evidence of positive results, although there was a plethora of secondary side effects that included increased tolerance, extreme psychological dependence and severe social disability.

On the other hand, fascinating research was being done in the area of neurochemistry and the effect of chemicals in the brain on mood, especially in regard to depression and its biochemical components. It was then that I began to ponder the question of the relationship between mood and food, and to question my professors of neuropharmacology, biochemistry and nutrition at the Harvard School of Public Health about it.

It seemed to me that my moods had an enormous impact

on my ability to diet, and I wanted to know why this was so and what could be done about it. Furthermore, I needed to maintain a strong energy level while I was losing weight. Medical school is not a spa, and a high degree of function is required. Because I needed to work hard and well, I paid close attention to how I felt after every meal.

There were some odd discoveries. For example, milk and yogurt were available on the hospital floor and I found that after snacking on them, I worked quite well for long periods of time. Chocolate bars, on the other hand, not only wreaked havoc with the calorie count, but left me (after an initial high) with an odd feeling of depression.

Using these personal discoveries, through trial and error I formulated a primitive version of what is now the Southampton Diet. I stayed on the diet for most of my four years of medical school, and by the time I graduated I had lost 210 pounds. Still, there was more to learn.

During my psychiatric residency at New York University I was faced with what is often called "the yo-yo problem"; that is, gaining five to fifteen pounds and then having to lose them again. Luckily, the university offered one of the finest psychopharmacology departments in the world, and it was there that I learned more about the biochemistry of the brain and how the brain may be affected by the food we eat. During this residency (a training process in which young doctors treat patients under the guidance of medical school professors), I also studied behavioral techniques. As I helped my patients apply these techniques to various emotional problems, I also tried them on myself, as aids to maintaining my weight loss.

Finally, I entered psychoanalysis—a requirement for the psychoanalytic practice I was planning at that time. Once again, my main concern was weight loss and, during the analysis, I probed for the psychological forces that bear on that problem.

You will find my conclusions, after these years of investigation, in this book—the refined Southampton Diet, specially structured for both those who must lose a great deal of weight and those who need only to lose five to twenty pounds.

What I had discovered was that the problem of weight loss is multifaceted and complex and will never respond to one single therapeutic approach. A thorough understanding of every aspect—medical, psychologic, biologic, nutritional and biochemical—is required, and only with that understanding was I able to structure a cure.

But the final result was personally gratifying in the most profound manner. Not only did I achieve the weight loss I had hoped for with little or no psychological stress, but I have maintained that loss ever since. The result of those years of study changed my life and, eventually, the lives of many of my patients.

You will read about some of these people later in the book. One of them—an orthopedic surgeon who found himself unable to operate because of his girth—returned to his practice to become one of the foremost orthopods in New York. Another, a dancer whose career was nearly destroyed by a ten-pound weight gain, has returned to her company and principal roles. Still another, a wealthy young woman whose obesity and lack of self-esteem had propelled her into an empty life peopled only with hangers-on who exploited her for her money, is happily married and an active sponsor of some of New York's most prestigious charity organizations.

The program I developed for myself and these patients is what you will read about in this book. Since, as I discovered, proper treatment of overweight requires more than one approach, I have devised a four-point program, as mentioned earlier. It consists of the following:

POINT ONE: The Diet

This is the ultimate medically and nutritionally sound diet.

You will live and eat normally while you are on it without carrying around a calorie counter or radically changing your lifestyle.

You can lose fifteen pounds in two weeks but you do not have to change this diet after two weeks. You can stay on it until you've lost all the weight you care to by using the second week's menus and instructions.

The Southampton Diet *always* works for *everyone*—and it works as quickly as the fad diets that have the potential for doing enormous harm to the body. And it works without counting calories because the diet itself does the counting for you!

As a physician, my ultimate responsibility is not to hurt anyone, not to allow anyone to get sick. "Above all," medical students are taught, "do no harm."

Furthermore, the diet is neither difficult nor exotic and does not require an extensive shopping list. It is pleasant, satisfying, stress-free and easy to follow. There are many menu variations, so one need never suffer a sense of deprivation or monotony, or hunger. You'll eat well. And you'll grow thin!

POINT TWO: The Fat Shield

The underlying causes of weight gain are psychological, and I have found that though these psychological factors may be diverse, they generally focus on one issue: negotiating feelings and relationships. The Fat Shield is that convenient method by which many of us remove ourselves from this anxiety-provoking problem. Yet, though this method is convenient, it is also self-destructive and self-punishing.

I will reshape your thinking and teach you *to stop punishing yourself*. When you've learned to do this, not only will you have conquered your compulsion to eat, but you'll enjoy what you do eat much more.

Dieting is never easy. It demands a certain kind of discipline and control. In order to achieve that discipline, you must first learn to experience the pleasure of doing something good for yourself and allow yourself the excitement and sense of euphoria that results from a healthy physical state.

You will learn to substitute *true* self-gratification for self-punishment. You will learn that you can lose weight without the negatives usually associated with weight loss, such as fatigue, crankiness or depression. You will experience the elation that comes from having achieved control of your own weight and mental balance.

POINT THREE: The Biochemical Miracle

Exciting new medical research shows a clear biochemical relationship between the food we eat and certain messages that are sent to our brains. These messages not only influence our moods but also affect our appetites.

I will show you how the chemicals in certain foods, or combination of foods, can affect your mind, often causing you to be less hungry or to eat more. You will also learn which foods are "happy" (in that they contribute to your happiness and self-esteem and truly satisfy your hunger) and which are "sad" (and may tend to depress you and actually make you hungrier).

The Southampton Diet itself is entirely new and revolutionary in this regard. It has been carefully refined to take into account the latest biochemical research being developed at major academic centers around the country.

I will explain in detail the influence of certain foods on your mind so that diet will be easier and more successful than you ever imagined possible. When you learn how this link between mood and food actually works, you will have no trouble at all dieting.

POINT FOUR: Behavioral Techniques for the Southampton Dieter

The success of the Southampton Diet for my patients has been extraordinary. Some—who needed to lose fifty, sixty or seventy pounds—lost as much as twenty pounds in two weeks. The average patient, whose goal was a ten- or twelve-pound loss, dropped those extra pounds in two to three weeks.

In my practice as well as in my own life, I found that one needs to be reminded that he or she is on a diet. In other words, it's sometimes easy to respond to the pressures of the moment and get sidetracked.

For this reason I have developed a series of mental programs that you can use when you need them. You will find them amazingly effective in allowing you to remember exactly what your goal is.

With these four life-changing points, I guarantee that this will be the last diet book you'll ever have to buy. You will lose as much weight as you want to and—equally as important—you'll keep the weight off.

2

WHY THE SOUTHAMPTON DIET WORKS—WHERE OTHERS HAVE FAILED

THE LATEST REPORTS ON OBESITY in the United States indicate that the average citizen weighs eighteen percent more than his or her recommended weight. Furthermore, in spite of the dozens of diet books on the market, the rate of obesity among Americans is increasing.

If so many of us are dieting so conscientiously, why are we getting fatter? Why do those who do manage to lose weight on diets gain it all back (and sometimes even more) before a year has passed? Why is the diet failure rate as high as ninety-five percent?

Obviously, there is no one answer to this question. It is a multifaceted problem and an interdisciplinary approach —that is, one that incorporates medical, psychiatric and nutritional understanding—is required.

From that moment in my late teens when I weighed 420 pounds and made up my mind to lose over 200 of them, I have continuously studied the field of weight loss. What I learned through these various institutions—Tufts Medical School, the Harvard School of Public Health and New York University—as well as in my own psychiatric practice is that though there is no one answer to overweight, the problem *can* be solved forever, using the results of medical and scientific research that are now available. This information forms the core of the program presented here.

The four points in the Southampton Diet plan provide you with the life-changing elements that have been missing from the diet plans you may have tried in the past. Let's examine each one of these points and see why this is so.

POINT ONE: The Diet Itself

To begin with, the Southampton Diet is medically and nutritionally sound, and you can remain on it until you've lost all the weight you need to.

Proper nutrition is crucial to dieting in many more ways than you can image, not the least of which is your actual *ability* to diet; that is, the level of your appetite. In other words, a poorly balanced diet is not only unhealthy but can actually hinder the weight loss process itself. This happens because your body starved of the nutrients it requires and naturally striving for life and health (a *homeostasis*, in medical terminology) then often demands twice as much food as it really needs, simply to make up for the deprivation. An unfortunate, self-defeating cycle! Not at all a program of weight loss, but, in the long run, one of weight *gain*. Forced into an unhealthy fad diet, your body can actually fight your desire and intention to lose weight.

Besides making the dieting process even more difficult than it already is, fad diets can do irreparable physical harm. The American public has been subject to a series of such diets in the past ten years, all of them presenting some

31

magical, off-balance cure. These hopeless schemes propose everything from watermelon to enzymes to "all the steak you can eat" as their fantasy formulas.

But fantasy formulas are often truly dangerous. At their best they can only be maintained for a few weeks, and at their worst they can cause serious damage to your heart, kidneys and other vital organs. In some extreme cases, they are even the cause of death.

Let's examine for a moment the fashionable notion of *ketosis*, which results from any of the low carbohydrate diets.

Ketosis is actually a starvationlike state in the body. The body is depleted of its normal fuel and substitutes for this fuel the protein contained in muscle tissue and vital organs. In this process, the body produces acid materials known as *ketones*. Some of these ketones pass out of the body through the urine, others enter the bloodstream and are used as fuel. Eventually, even the brain, normally fueled by glucose, draws most of its energy from ketones. This is actually, by definition, a state of starvation.

Supposing that, in your desperation to lose weight, you were foolish enough to embark on one of these diets, willing even to risk the possibility of debilitating fatigue, a drop in blood pressure, dizziness, kidney damage and potential birth defects—would you lose weight?

Initially, it may appear so. But the fact of the matter is that the weight loss through ketosis consists mainly of water, not fat. Low carbohydrate–high protein diets cause the kidneys to flush sodium out of the body. Sodium is what permits the body to retain water. As the sodium level drops, your body loses water (and can, incidentally, easily become dehydrated).

The results of these diet programs are almost inevitable. Few of them dare claim that you should stay on the plan more than a couple of weeks, so (I certainly hope) you soon go back to a more balanced diet. The minute you do that, sodium is restored to your body and the "water weight" returns.

Nothing could be further from this miserable yo-yo routine than the Southampton Diet program. But I have seen the results of this depressing and dangerous cycle when patients who have been subjected to these diets come to my office for help.

Madeline was one such patient. She was nineteen years old, five feet six inches tall, and weighed 235 pounds when she first walked into my office in Southampton. The last time her weight had been normal was at age eleven, and she had gained 120 pounds since that time. She had thick, dark hair and lovely violet eyes that reminded me of the actress Elizabeth Taylor, who, incidentally, must also deal with problems of overweight. But, unlike Taylor, whose weight difficulties developed later in life, Madeline's weight gain began when she was a youngster, and her problem was much more severe.

Though she was exceedingly wealthy and could easily afford an extensive wardrobe, she cloaked her shame in baggy blue jeans and a series of African overblouses cut for men. For the past three years Madeline had sought help from one doctor after another in her attempt to lose at least a hundred pounds. Some of the physicians had prescribed diet pills (amphetamines) on which she had indeed lost thirty or forty pounds, only to find that when she stopped taking these dangerous drugs, she gained fifty pounds within a few weeks. In other forays, she was given thyroid pills, water pills or liquid protein—all with the same result.

Madeline's last dieting attempt had brought her to the author of a famous "ketonic" two-week diet. While on this diet she had indeed lost weight (although, she reported, she'd felt extremely ill during the whole period), but three weeks later she gained back all the weight *plus* another fifteen pounds.

By this time, poor Madeline had reached a weight of 235

pounds and in utter desperation had gone to a surgeon who stapled her stomach. ("Stapling" is an unconscionable procedure in which the lumen, or center, of the stomach is made smaller so that less food can be held in it.) The result of this hideous operation was that Madeline simply continued to eat as before and then disgorged the food she had eaten by vomiting. The vomiting, in turn, depleted the electrolyte content in her body to the point where she had to be rushed to the hospital for intravenous potassium feedings in order to save her life.

As ghastly as this may sound, it is still not the end of the story. When, under my guidance, Madeline was referred to a hospital for surgical removal of the staples, adhesions were found on her stomach wall—the result of poor surgery. Those adhesions cause her chronic pain to this day.

Few of us, thank goodness, would allow ourselves to be driven to such extremes—even by the desire to lose weight. But the emotional stresses behind Madeline's weight problem are not totally beyond our understanding.

Madeline's mother was an extremely beautiful, socially prominent and wealthy woman who cared a good deal about her own stunning good looks, as well as Madeline's, of course. Madeline's father, whom she adored, had left her mother and had continued, throughout his extremely high-powered, Wall-Street-centered life, to focus most of his attention on beautiful women. When he remarried (another stunning partner) he wanted little involvement with his first family and, in fact, lost interest. Madeline continued to live with her mother, spending her summers and weekends in their large Georgian home at the beach. But she never participated in the whirl of parties her mother enjoyed.

Madeline was angry at both her mother, whom she blamed for the divorce, and her father, for his neglect of her. Since both her parents valued physical beauty and wanted her to be thin and attractive, Madeline was able to use the weapon of her own weight gain against both of them. She was so successful in this vengeful battle that her father, disgusted with his daughter's 235-pound appearance, refused to speak to her for two years.

What a cost to Madeline! And how depressed and anxious she was.

Yet from the first day that this distressed young woman came into my office until several months later, when she had achieved exactly the weight she aimed for—130 pounds—her spirits began to lift.

This in spite of the fact that I immediately told her that her first task was to recognize she *could not* lose 105 pounds in five weeks, but that in a systematic, wholesome fashion, she would lose it over a period of time—approximately 25 weeks. She quickly found that since the Southampton Diet is not only nutritionally healthy but includes a special balance of mood-controlling foods, her state of mind was actually changing as the dieting process progressed. (You will read about these foods—one of the most significant discoveries for dieters in the past half-century—at a further point.)

As Madeline began to steadily and systematically lose weight, her visible anger and resentment soon gave way to a cheerful, hopeful, positive attitude. Furthermore, her attitudes about herself and dieting went through a profound and extensive change, which can best be described by Point Two of the Southampton Diet.

POINT TWO: The Fat Shield

I will describe the formation and results of the Fat Shield in some detail in the next chapter. Let me say here only that it is an unconscious mechanism by which

many of us "shield" ourselves from the necessity of negotiating what may be anxiety-producing relationships. Once
having established that protection, however, we are often
defeated in our attempts to renegotiate—that is, further
relationships, more often than not sexual ones, become
even more difficult, and we tend to conclude that we are
helpless to do anything about this situation.

If there is any one psychological factor that I have found
most inevitably present in a person with a weight-loss problem, it is a sense of helplessness. I remember very well my
own feeling, before that turning point in Paris, that my
overweight and the isolated lifestyle that accompanied it
were inevitable, and that I was doomed to this hateful state
for life.

This perception—or rather, misperception—was precisely at the heart of Madeline's difficulties with dieting,
and you may find some trace of it in your mind as well.

When you believe that your mind and body are beyond
your ability to control them, you are caught in an awful
trap. I know this sense of helplessness very well because
before that turning point in my own life, when I began
what has evolved into the Southampton Diet program, I
was thoroughly immersed in it myself. One does not, after
all, expand to a weight of 420 pounds without severe mental distress, and one does not lose 210 pounds without a
complete change in mental patterns.

In Madeline's case, all four points of the Southampton
Diet program were essential, but we began by disputing this
concept of helplessness.

How had it come about?

Well, of course this young woman had some emotional
difficulties in her relationship with her parents. She also
had problems negotiating friendships. (Madeline was the
wealthy young woman I spoke of in the last chapter who
was exploited for her money.) But we all face emotional

hurdles of one kind or another and self-destruction will not help us clear them.

What Madeline needed to realize—and she did this readily—was that the tack she had taken was, in fact, self-destructive and had led directly to her feelings of helplessness. Furthermore, there was a direct connection between Madeline's state of mind (her *mood*, as we refer to it sometimes) and her appetite.

The Southampton Diet program is the first and only weight-loss plan to describe this precise dynamic . . . the discovery that mental equilibrium, a happy state of mind, almost always controls the appetite while the opposite—a sense of lethargy or depression—increases it.

In Madeline's case, fad dieting had actually *increased* her sense of helplessness and, inevitably, her appetite . . . as it usually does for most of us.

Suppose, for example, that a certain fad diet is extremely austere, depriving you of either variety or pleasure in eating. What will happen?

You will soon go off it. You will begin to feel deprived, resentful and put-upon. You will not tolerate this deprivation for long and you will soon begin your old eating pattern again.

Suppose the diet is nutritionally unsound, as most invariably are. You will experience fatigue and lethargy; you may even find the level of your accomplishment dropping. Since our competitive world demands that each of us produce at a substantial rate, you will come to the conclusion that you simply cannot afford to be tired and undernourished, and you will soon go off that diet as well.

You will also go off your diet if you're deprived of the important new biochemical discovery—the mood/food connection, which will be described in detail in Chapter 4 —that only the Southampton Diet offers; that is, the control of your mood, and therefore your will to diet, through

37

a specially balanced intake of foods that contain amino acids along with the nutrients that help them work.

In short, you'll go off your diet if it is not specially orchestrated to permit you to *remain* on it—as I did—until you've lost all the weight you care to.

But here's the next crucial consideration. When you do go off one of these fad diets, the inevitable result is an emotionally damaging one: a sense of failure. Obviously, no one feels *good* about having failed at a task they've set for themselves; failure never produces an "up" positive mood. What we are generally left with is a sense of helplessness which works in classic psychological tandem with depression, the sense of impotence feeding depression and vice versa.

When you read the next chapter in this book, you will find an explanation of the effects of moods of joy or sadness on your appetite. Let's just say here that depression, whether minimal or severe, changes one's appetite, more often than not increasing it. We can easily see, then, how fad diets may very well have led you, as they did Madeline, to a sense of helplessness and an increased appetite. No wonder they haven't been successful!

Once Madeline realized the extent to which she had actually permitted this self-punishment to continue, she was well on her way to a substantial weight loss and eventually made a brilliant new life for herself. In fact she phoned me about a year later to tell me she was marrying a young architect whom she had met at one of her mother's parties!

Phyllis, another patient, is a good example of how the mood/food connection works in less extreme cases of overweight. Phyllis, the thirty-one-year-old wife of a Southampton lawyer, was the mother of two children, one a four-month-old baby. She was tall (five feet nine inches), blond and well respected in the community for her charming fund-raising galas in behalf of local artists. Her husband, whose practice was extensive, spent ten or eleven hours a day at the office and often brought home work to do over the weekend. Because of her husband's heavy work load, Phyllis told me, there were times when she felt neglected.

After the birth of her second child, Phyllis had experienced a mild postpartum depression. She was not incapacitated and she accomplished what she needed to do around the house. But, she told me when she visited the office, "I just can't seem to get *up* to running those affairs anymore. I keep having to push myself to make those phone calls."

Coincidentally, since the birth of her last child, Phyllis had been about fourteen pounds overweight.

This young housewife and mother had always been athletic, conscious of her weight and able to lose the two or three pounds she occasionally gained with no problem at all. She was much too sensible a person ever to subject herself to a fad diet, but she could not understand why she was unable to regain the eating pattern that had worked so well for her before the baby was born.

Although Phyllis's mild depression was not *caused* by a fad diet, it does present a clear example of how a healthy, well-integrated, sensitive and caring person can respond to a sense of helplessness. Feeling that she was impotent in her attempts at weight loss and without control over what she ate, she attempted to assuage this miserable feeling with a particular passion of hers—chocolate éclairs!

If we stop and think of what we all know about the effects of sugar on the body, we can imagine what this sweet pacifier did to Phyllis. As we all do, she experienced a sudden "rush" as the glucose surged through her digestive system and then, about ten minutes later, a "letdown." This rush, followed by a letdown, is how glucose always acts on the body, and in Phyllis's case that "down" feeling simply reinforced the depression and sense of helplessness that were already operating on her psyche. And led her to eat another éclair, of course!

The Southampton Diet program was a very simple answer for Phyllis.

From time to time, most of us experience mild feelings of depression that often go hand in hand with that sense of helplessness. When Phyllis recognized that syndrome, she could immediately see that she was not helpless at all. Quite the opposite! Her brain played a trick on her, and all that was needed was to reverse this trick.

As soon as Phyllis began to eat the foods prescribed in the diet, what she had misperceived as a state of helplessness vanished. She was soon totally in control of both what she ate and the numbers on her scale.

In short, the depression/helplessness/fat cycle went into a speedy reverse. Phyllis's mood lightened and the fourteen pounds she had gained melted off easily. She was soon back at her community work, helping to make the Hamptons as buoyantly creative as ever.

Was Phyllis's happy mood change merely the result of her change in perception? Emphatically not.

An important factor is a totally new biochemical consideration that has never before been incorporated into a diet plan. That is the third point on the Southampton Diet plan.

POINT THREE: The Biochemical Miracle—Mood and Food

This vital discovery will be explained in detail in Chapter 4. Specifically, the connection involves the latest scientific analyses of the powerful effects of amino acids on the brain.

Recent studies have shown that thin people, that is, those who have *no* weight problems, eat mainly in response to true hunger. Those who *do* have weight problems eat in response to other signals from the brain. What causes the brain to issue those signals to so many of us who have difficulty with what we call our "appetites"? There is strong scientific evidence to suggest that amino acids play an amazing contributory role (through a process I'll describe later). What is even more remarkable, especially in light of the fact that other diet programs have never taken this into account, is that almost *all* these important amino acids can only reach our brain through the food we eat!

This mood/food connection is one of the main features of the Southampton Diet program. I am thoroughly convinced, both through my own experience and that of my patients, that the specific balance of the amino acids in our diet affects our moods and, therefore, our appetites and ability to diet. My own belief in this biochemical reaction is so strong that I have compiled a list of what I regard as "happy" and "sad" foods, which you will find in Chapter 5.

Just one example from the hundreds of people whose weight problems were solved through Southampton Diet's control of this biochemical action is Bradford, a middle-aged orthopedic surgeon whose extra weight had settled heavily around his waistline.

As a physician, Bradford knew better than to subject himself to crash diets. Instead, he had been attending weekly meetings in New York City sponsored by a large and basically responsible weight-loss workshop. According to the rules of this particular workshop, participants were issued a card on which was stamped their theoretical weight loss for the week. At each meeting they were required to record their actual weight loss next to the theoretical one and present this data to the group.

On Bradford's first visit to the office, he showed me his card. According to what was written there, he had actually *gained* sixty pounds over the five-month period during which he attended the meetings. He then confessed that his midsection had become so cumbersome that he could not get a complete view of the surgical procedure and couldn't handle a scalpel properly. This is such a terrible state for an orthopedic surgeon to find himself in that Bradford had been referring all his patients to another physician.

Now it is undoubtedly true that Bradford did, as he insisted, find the group method of weight loss somewhat embarrassing. But even more important, to my mind, were his debilitating mood swings. As he reported it, they varied from day to day, hour to hour, changing after a meal or a snack (and snacking was something he found himself doing more and more often). His moods ranged from a heavy lethargy that made it difficult for him to get out of bed in the morning, to a hyperirascibility, expressed in a snappish irritation with the nurses and aides at the hospital. He was, by the time he came to my office, highly suspicious of *any* diet program and cynical in his outlook on life and his own ability to continue in his practice as an orthopedic surgeon.

Bradford was willing, however, to give losing weight one more try. So he and I made a pact. It was one that is exactly the same as the contract you will find in Chapter 8. He promised me that he would give the Southampton Diet program a two-week trial.

Three days after Bradford began the program, I received a phone call from his office.

"The very first day on the diet was difficult," he said, "but the second was not so hard, and the third miraculously easy."

I had discussed my belief in the effect of amino acids with Bradford on his first visit and now, he said, he was convinced of its importance. By the second day on the diet, he reported, his mood swings had completely disappeared. He was feeling happy, cheerful and positively hopeful about his future. In retrospect, he felt that his snacking and overeating had been due to his attempt to assuage his irritability and depressed feelings.

By the end of the first week, Bradford weighed in at my office with an eleven-pound loss, and by the end of the second week, he had shed twenty pounds. Eventually he lost all of the seventy-five pounds we felt was necessary for him.

Bradford and I became close friends over those weeks and had many long and fascinating discussions about my theory and the powerful effects of amino acids on mood and appetite. It was Bradford, among several other friends and colleagues, who prevailed upon me to write this book.

POINT FOUR: Behavioral Techniques for the Southampton Diet

The mood/food connection is an important part of the Southampton Diet, yet there is still another point that it necessary to a diet program. No matter how well our moods and, therefore, our appetites are controlled, most of us (though not Bradford!) sometimes simply forget we're on a diet. Sometimes, under the stress of daily living, pressures on the job or in our relationships with lovers or friends, we lose sight of our goal.

This is a serious stumbling block in any long-range dieting program and it is the final reason for the failure of most diet plans. My solution to this problem is a series of mental maneuvers that I have developed over the years for myself and my patients. These mental maneuvers are actually behavioral replacement techniques, which help you form the new habits that will assure your being thin and happy forever.

One patient who made particularly good use of some of

these techniques was Alicia, a young fashion photographer who generally summered as a member of a "share"—a common arrangement in the Hamptons, in which a specified number of single people rent rooms in a house for the season.

Alicia was lively and chic and loved the Hamptons. ("I would *die* if I couldn't get out here on the weekends," she told me.) But every summer, she found that by Labor Day she had gained five to ten pounds. She disliked returning to the city and to her work with her fashionable clothing strained across her hips and waist, which was where, she explained, those added few pounds always settled.

When I questioned Alicia about her eating habits, she told me that the group of single people she lived with usually ate together in the dining room of the rented house. "We kind of gobble our food, I guess," she said, "because we're always in a hurry to get to the beach or to a party." Then she laughed and added, "Whereupon I eat even more there!"

The first week of the Southampton Diet brought Alicia's weight quickly down to her normal 118 pounds, but because it was important for her to maintain that weight, I suggested the following:

"When you sit down at the table with your friends, pretend that you're in a competition—not to see who can eat the most the fastest, but who can eat the slowest. Try to be the *last* to put down your fork. And," I added, "it *is* a good idea to eat something before you go to a party. That way you won't be so hungry that you gobble your food. But if it's a dinner party, make sure that you eat only the snacks that are prescribed on the Southampton Diet before you go. And let me know how this works out."

I received a call from Alicia in my New York office just after Labor Day of that year.

"Hallelujah!" she bubbled. "It worked! I didn't gain

weight this summer. This time I came back with energy, a great suntan and not one extra pound."

You will find more of these behavioral techniques in Chapter 7. Most of my patients have found them extremely helpful. Furthermore, I have used every one of them at one time or another, either to lose the 210 pounds or to maintain my current healthy weight, and I can guarantee that they work.

Before you turn to Chapter 7, however, you should learn about the psychological forces that lead to weight gain and how the Southampton Diet circumvents these forces.

3

THE FAT SHIELD—YOUR
WORST ENEMY

THE BASIC CAUSES OF OVERWEIGHT—whether 2 or 200 pounds—are almost always psychological. We can, if we wish, define and categorize each of these psychic factors ("affects," as psychiatrists often refer to them), and undoubtedly find traces of every known emotional conflict.

But research of this nature would, I believe, prove valueless.

In the first place, overweight people are not mentally ill and there is no reason, per se, for most of them to spend long hours and a great deal of money on psychotherapy. If, indeed, psychotherapy is indicated or desired, I believe it should be separate from the weight-loss process.

In the second place, what is really needed is an understanding of *how* we gain weight (that is, the "dynamic") and *how we can reverse this process.*

Understanding how you have constructed what I call "the Fat Shield"—and *everyone* who is overweight, even if only by a few pounds, has one—is absolutely necessary if you are to take full advantage of the Southampton Diet.

46

The diet itself provides a lifetime change in your eating habits so you need never begin the process again. But to utilize it fully, you must be aware of the psychological roots of the problem.

What I have learned—both from my own experience in losing 210 pounds and from my patients—has led me to the following conclusions:

Whatever the basic cause of overeating, and whether or not this problem has been solved, it soon becomes less important to the psyche than the fact that the person is already fat (or fatter than he or she wants to be).

That is, the condition of being overweight itself creates certain emotional stresses that are usually just as damaging to one's sense of self as whatever caused the eating problem in the first place.

Put still another way: Fat itself is destructive to the ego.

How we embark on this self-punishing dynamic is quite simple. The very first time we eat something in response to an emotional urge—rather than simple hunger—we begin a pattern that eventually takes on a life of its own, quite apart from the original emotion. This pattern is the inner structure of the Fat Shield—an unfortunate mechanism that "protects" us from closeness, sexuality or intimacy.

It originates in the following manner:

Suppose, for example, that as a child you were either forbidden to have something extremely important to you (a bicycle, perhaps) or were frightened by a certain social situation (such as a cabin full of strangers at summer camp). Suppose, as well, that in either of these situations you were offered a box of cookies at the same time. If you ate those cookies, you might have felt an immediate sense of relief and gratification. There is no question that for many people oral stimulation provides quick solace for emotional distress.

The relief, of course, is momentary. The situation that

upset you would not have changed. Eating those cookies would not bring you the bicycle or magically transform your cabinmates into old familiar buddies. But the first step in structuring a potential Fat Shield would have been taken. Food would have been used to quickly (and most superficially) assuage emotional distress.

In my own case, this pattern began as a response to my anger at my grandmother. In reality, eating cookies or lasagna did not remove me from her care, but the self-punishing dynamic (oral solace for emotional stress) was slowly and steadily imprinted on my preconscious mind.

This is the pattern that plagues most of us who are overweight. We have learned to respond to psychic discomfort with an oral "pacifier" and we continue that response even though the original cause (the fear of cabinmates, the anger at a parent or whatever it may be) no longer exists. Only this inner structure and the resultant overweight remains. (Or, in what is commonly described as the "seesaw" or "yo-yo" effect, the added weight reappears under a variety of stress conditions.)

Not only, in fact, does the Fat Shield remain, but it is perpetuated and increased in a particularly devilish manner.

Being fat creates its *own* emotional distress. As "fatties" we perceive ourselves (often correctly) as less appealing to other people. We then become more isolated, less inclined to pursue intimate relationships with others.

But—and this is the diabolical part of the dynamic—as any person withdraws from intimacy and closeness, he or she becomes prone to one of the greatest inducements to overeating—a strong sense of deprivation, emptiness and, eventually, depression.

In short, overweight leads to depression. And depression, in turn, leads to more overweight. No wonder that most of the patients enter the door of my office with an intense feeling of helplessness. They are caught in a cruel self-punishing trap.

These Southampton residents are, for the most part, handsome, accomplished and motivated people who live and work in a glamorous but highly competitive world. They are confronted, almost daily, with nerve-wracking situations—theatrical performances, auditions, exhibits, business deals often involving millions of dollars. Most of us must face difficult situations in our busy lives. To find ourselves, under these conditions, with the added stress produced by extra pounds is quite intolerable.

The Southampton Diet program is specially designed to contradict the sense of helplessness and immediately remove us from this trap.

Sarah, one of my patients, is a particularly good example of how the program accomplishes this, because both the desire to lose weight and the destructive patterning factors were so strong in her case.

A pretty thirty-two-year-old with long brown hair, Sarah was an articles editor of a national women's fashion magazine. This soft-spoken young woman came to my office directly from the intensive care unit of a New York hospital. She had been hospitalized after several weeks on a popular diet that consisted mainly of fruit. Prior to her hospitalization, Sarah had not only failed to achieve the twelve-pound loss she had hoped for on this diet, but had found herself behaving in a hyper, erratic manner. When she phoned the diet's author, she had been advised to eat still more fruit.

This sort of foolish diet depletes the body of potassium (among other nutrients) and is actually life-threatening. After four days in intensive care, Sarah was understandably frightened and unsure of herself.

Still, she remained anxious to lose weight. She was a fashionable, gregarious young woman and wanted very much to take part in the whirl of parties and dating that surrounds the publishing world in Manhattan. Sarah's family physician was not sympathetic to her desire to lose those extra pounds, she told me. It was merely a "cosmetic" problem, he insisted.

But Sarah was unable to lose those few pounds on her own, and when she came into my office, her wide hazel eyes were on the verge of tears.

"I don't want to do anything crazy again," she half-whispered, "but I feel awful when I weigh this much, and I don't know what to do about it."

Sarah was telling me what I had heard from many other patients—that she felt helpless. A sense of helplessness, as we have seen, is usually an indication of depression, the sort of mild, nonvegetative depression that often afflicts high achievers.

With Sarah, as with most of my overweight patients, I made no attempt to probe for the deep psychological conflicts that might be buried in her unconscious mind. She was certainly not someone I would characterize as mentally ill, nor even highly neurotic. Her discomfort with her social life and her failure to lose weight were both feeding heavily into her sense of helplessness. These were the problems that had to be attacked immediately.

After listening to Sarah for a while, I asked her just one question: "Are you ready to begin a diet designed to support a healthy life?"

When her answer was an unequivocal "Yes," we began immediately on the Southampton Diet program.

Obviously, Sarah, like any other overweight person, had *some* underlying conflicts or she wouldn't have gained the weight. But I believe that any analytic work on those problems—if desired by the patient—should be separate from the dieting process.

What *is* effective, and was certainly so in Sarah's case, is a program that organizes your life so that you can develop a certain diet lifestyle. As Sarah began the program, she found, as you will, that she was eating specific foods at specific times, organizing her eating habits through breakfast, lunch, dinner and snacks, and removing choices and options. This was, for her, the beginning of a lifetime change.

In other words, Sarah began the Southampton Diet even though she was feeling blue. *Then,* as her systematic weight loss progressed, her *self-esteem* rose and she was soon dashing happily about to the publishing parties and galas she enjoyed so much. She was also able to handle many of the problems that had previously plagued her, not the least of which were those patterning habits I spoke of earlier.

Sarah's eating pattern was clearly a direct outgrowth of her home environment: a close-knit ethnic family in which love and warmth were expressed through the offering of food. Every member of the family was plump and none of them saw any reason why Sarah shouldn't be satisfied with this extra padding as well. But whereas the other members of the family lived within a small ethnic community in one of New York's other boroughs, Sarah was making her life and her career in the larger, more fashionable world of Manhattan.

On one of her visits to the office, I asked her how she had handled that problem.

"I called a meeting," she answered brightly, "at the dinner table. As soon as the whole family was there, I just issued a proclamation. I told them that it was extremely important for me to lose weight and that I intended to do just that."

I must admit that I laughed at the image of this formal proceeding over the family dinner table.

"Did they understand why?" I asked.

"Not a bit," Sarah replied. "They all just sat there, wide-eyed, looking at me as if I had gone bananas. But then they said, 'Okay.' And nobody has bothered me about eating ever since."

Obviously, though her motivation was incomprehensible to them, Sarah's family regarded her happiness as a high priority. But it was Sarah's clear understanding of how her Fat Shield had been structured that allowed her to communicate her needs so effectively.

Sarah, like most of my patients, really *knew* subconsciously what she had been doing to herself by gaining weight. Most of us who find ourselves caught in this depressing cycle are at least partially aware of it. What is required to interrupt the cycle is: 1) to admit it to our full awareness, as I did in that awful moment in the Opéra in Paris when I could not fit in my seat; 2) to understand the dynamic of the Fat Shield fully; and 3) most important, to embark on a diet that will ultimately and finally assure us of being thin and happy for the rest of our lives.

As Sarah found, the Southampton Diet is exactly that program. But her thorough awareness of the inner structure of her own Fat Shield was what assured her of staying on the diet so consistently.

Not everyone, after all, immediately reaches for food when he or she is confronted with stress. Those of us who have been patterned in this manner must learn how damaging it is to our well-being, how food consumed under these conditions is, metaphorically speaking, poison to our systems.

I can think of no more poignant evidence of the emotional punishment inflicted by this dynamic than was presented by a patient I'll call Patti.

Patti was seventeen years old, the daughter of a diplomatic family, a talented ballet dancer who had won a scholarship to one of the major ballet schools in New York. I was informed by the ballet teacher who recommended Patti to my care that she had been highly rated at the various schools she had attended.

As lovely as Patti was, however (she had beautiful long legs and exquisite carriage), she found when she reached New York that she was simply one among many equally talented and lovely young dancers. Frightened by this sudden competition, she attempted to assuage her anxieties by oral gratification. She found herself stopping every day on her way to classes and, as she described it to me, "pigging out" on croissants and other pastries in the bakery near school.

Overweight is, of course, the ultimate bane of ballet dancers and the ruination of many careers. At five feet five-and-a-half inches and 135 pounds, Patti's dance career was in real jeopardy. Over a period of four months, since she had first arrived in New York, she had constructed a thirty-pound Fat Shield. Its evidence was to be seen not only in the roundness of her body, but in the dullness of her eyes. She was quite straightforward when expressing her problem.

"I'm depressed," she said. "I can't help it. That's just how I feel."

"Are you aware, Patti," I asked, "that overeating—particularly the wrong foods—can actually *lead* to depression, and that the depression, in its turn, can cause you to overeat?"

She hadn't quite thought of it that way, she admitted.

You have read about the effects of depression on the appetite in the last chapter, but because it is so important to the renewable nature of the Fat Shield, let's examine it in more detail here.

Depression, whether mild or extreme, is characterized by a drop in motivation, mobility and sociability. A depressed person tends to be less available to others and quite sedentary, which provides him or her with little to do but eat. This is the reason why you gain weight when you're on vacation or on a cruise. There's often nothing much else to do but eat!

Furthermore, as we've seen, even mild depression affects the appetite, either increasing or decreasing it.

If a person is already overweight when the "low" mood strikes, he or she rarely *loses* their appetite. The tendency is almost *always* to eat more and gain more. Thus the Fat Shield renews itself.

Patti listened carefully to this explanation and then nodded her head thoughtfully. What I had described, she admitted, was exactly what had been happening to her.

"The Southampton Diet is designed to interrupt this cycle," I told her, "but you must decide yourself if you really want to break the pattern."

Unlike some of my patients, Patti did not agree immediately. Although, as a psychiatrist, I could make many conjectures about her initial indecision, it would really be of no value, nor would psychotherapy have been the answer. Patti's depression/eating cycle had to be interrupted by her own choice. The Southampton Diet, which is specially orchestrated to provide nutrition and mood elevation, was available to her. But she had to make that commitment.

Indeed, she finally did. Several weeks later, Patti appeared at my office. She was ready to begin, she said. The pain of those extra pounds and all they implied had finally impressed itself on her consciousness and she was determined to end the self-punishment. She embarked on the Southampton Diet, and within a week she had lost seven pounds.

"How do you feel?" I asked her.

"I feel like a dancer," she said, and added, "again."

In Patti's case her Fat Shield had been "protecting" her from her career. In many other cases, it "protects" us from relationships. Many of the patients I see in Southampton are recently separated or divorced. Often they are wary of entering into new relationships and their weight gain is an unconscious mechanism that enables them to avoid those relationships.

I doubt that you need to be convinced that being encased in an excess layer of fat is, in fact, depressing. Nor are you unaware that most people in our society regard being overweight as unattractive, nor that they respond in a negative manner to those whom they regard as unattractive.

Should further proof be needed, however, a number of recent studies at universities across the country on the effects of human appearance have led to the following conclusions:

Physically attractive people are not only regarded as more poised, sensitive, sexually warm, sincere, interesting and successful than others but they are also given preferential treatment. Dr. Ellen Berscheid, a professor of psychology at the University of Minnesota, has studied the effects of physical attractiveness for fifteen years. Physically unattractive youngsters should not assume that the difficulties they experience in school or with friends are the result of a low intelligence level, poor personality, or any character flaw, she told a *New York Times* reporter. According to her findings, the problems of unattractive children could well be the direct result of their looks.

In other words, it has now been proved that your physical appearance does indeed have a profound effect on your happiness and success in life. Fat people are not—in spite of the clichés to the contrary—happy people. The truth of the matter is that in our society they are usually isolated, lonely and depressed.

No one could be more aware of that fact than I was—at 210 pounds overweight.

The Southampton Diet provides the solution to that problem, but understanding the nature of the Fat Shield will assure you of avoiding any annoying "seesaw" effect of regaining and then having to lose the weight again.

It might also help you to be aware of what I describe as "the Euphoria Plateau." Dieting, we all know, requires a certain kind of discipline and control. And unlike the external controls applied by military training or a strict ballet mistress, the controls for dieting are internal and personal. In order to achieve those controls, you must allow yourself to experience the happiness that comes from doing something good for yourself—the self-gratification of success, the joy of fulfillment, the excitement of good health. It is this positive sense of accomplishment that the Southampton Diet provides.

Oddly enough, however, buried within that state of fulfillment is one of those difficulties we encounter on the road to being thin and happy. It can occur any time between the third or fourth day and the second week of any successful dieting attempt.

Diana was one patient who found herself in the Euphoria Plateau. She learned to use it to her advantage, and perhaps her experience will help you as well.

Diana was a forty-year-old mother of two active youngsters, one ten years old and the other twelve and a half. She was a tall, outgoing, assertive woman who had left a promising career as a producer of television commercials to marry and raise her two children. Diana enjoyed her life as a wife and mother and particularly loved spending her summers on her large farm outside Southampton. She had no regrets about leaving her career. Her only complaint was that in the past few years she had been unable to keep her originally svelte 130-pound figure, in spite of the fact that she was an avid equestrian and spent many hours a day riding her horses.

Diana came to the Southampton Diet with little hope for the sort of success she wanted. She didn't believe in diets, she said, though *not* because she had been unable to lose a substantial portion of her fifteen-pound goal while on them. The problem was, as she put it: "What will I weigh in a month?"

In other words, Diana had been living with the seesaw problem. She felt that her past attempts at dieting had been failures either because she'd never quite reached her goal or because she'd never maintained the weight loss for more than a week or so.

Nevertheless, she was willing to try one more time, and when she arrived at my office for her second appointment (one week after she began the diet), she had successfully dropped six of the fifteen pounds she intended to lose. Like most of us who break the fat cycle, she was feeling excited, cheery and a bit superior. She had it "knocked," she reported. She was in control and she felt terrific.

"Have you ever felt this way before while dieting?" I asked. Diana thought for a moment and then, with an embarrassed smile, recalled that she had, though perhaps to a lesser extent. This euphoria had appeared several times in the past, usually within the first week of a diet.

Now, let me assure you immediately that a sense of buoyancy and well-being is entirely appropriate on the Southampton Diet. In fact, the diet itself, through both psychological and biochemical means, is designed to give you precisely that feeling. But, as I told Diana, what you must watch out for is what you *do* with that feeling.

Do not use it as an excuse to go off the diet!

When Diana recalled her previous attempts at dieting, she realized that she had usually felt a strong sense of superiority and accomplishment at some time during the first week. The problem was that she had drawn from that state of euphoria the mistaken conclusion that she had nothing more to conquer.

This is the only warning to be issued regarding the Euphoria Plateau you may experience on the Southampton Diet: This plateau should not be regarded as an end point of your efforts. Learn to read it, as Diana soon did, as a state of mind specially engineered to help you in your steady progress toward your goal of being forever-thin. It is only the first of many rewards. You will earn many more social and career successes in your new, happy life.

When Diana realized how she had misinterpreted this signal, she quickly put it into proper perspective. This time she used her happy, self-confident state of mind to continue on the diet until she was able to reach and maintain her goal. At her last visit, she reported that her weight had fluctuated no more than four pounds over the past six months.

The Euphoria Plateau that Diana had experienced is undoubtedly even more pronounced in the Southampton Diet than in any others, because mental well-being is exactly what the diet is designed to produce. The fact that the mind and body are inextricably linked has long been accepted in psychosomatic medicine. We know that emotions are usually accompanied by some physical response; fear by perspiration and increased heartbeat, anger by a rise in blood pressure and so on. There is certainly no reason to assume that appetite is not affected by our state of mind as well. For the first time, however, this diet actually identifies *the state of mind that promotes dieting as well as the one that doesn't.*

Emotional equilibrium, we have seen, is the fundamental concept behind the Southampton Diet, and to achieve it you must be strongly committed to a program of what I call "Being Good to Yourself." Just as we have learned that the Fat Shield is really a form of self-punishment, a means of isolating ourselves from others, we must also learn what truly caring for ourselves actually means.

Shielding your body with fat is a cruel and unfair way to treat yourself in today's society. It is, as we have seen, destructive to the ego. It deals with the issues all of us must negotiate—love, intimacy, sex, being close—but it deals with them in a very self-destructive fashion. The Fat Shield creates a lonely, isolated, frustrated, depressed, frequently angry human being who rightly feels he or she is missing out on the world.

But what, then, is its opposite? What does being good to yourself entail? Does it mean going on a shopping spree and buying yourself a dress that is several sizes too large? Or buying the car that is not really the one you want but the one you can fit into with less discomfort?

My view of caring for yourself is as follows: keeping your body trim and healthy, creating positive self-esteem and a sense of identity. The desire to do this is natural—if sometimes unconscious—in every human being. The Southampton Diet plan involves cultivating, nourishing and strengthening this desire.

As you embark on this program, you will find, I hope, that you are asking yourself one particular question again and again. You may be about to take a walk, go to a movie or enter a pastry shop, and before you do any of these things, you will think: Is what I am about to do helping to *care for* or to *punish* myself?

As you progress on the diet, you will find that the *answers* to this question become infinitely clearer. You will know that punishing yourself means building a Fat Shield and caring for yourself means opening your life to success and happiness. You will discover, as Patti, Diana and the others you've read about here discovered, that the special nutri-

tional and biochemical balance provided by the diet promotes the state of fulfillment and health that will help you
answer that question. In the next chapter, you will learn
about the all-important biochemical balance. You will also
learn about the effect of amino acids on the brain and how,
for the first time, the Southampton Diet makes use of the
brilliant discoveries in this new field to insure your weight
loss.

4

THE BIOCHEMICAL MIRACLE—
MOOD AND FOOD

NEUROCHEMISTRY IS the result of what is unquestionably the greatest medical exploration of our time. The outgrowth of a twenty-five-year investigation, it has revolutionized psychiatry and provided the world with fantastic new drugs to treat all sorts of emotional disorders. These drugs range from tranquilizers and antidepressants to all manner of mood-altering chemicals that have cut the number of patients in our mental hospitals in half.

Furthermore, this brilliant medical breakthrough has enormously increased our understanding of how chemicals affect the brain; specifically, how chemicals affect mood.

What the Southampton Diet does, for the very first time, is to use all that has been learned about the biochemistry of the brain's smallest particles to make your mind work *for* you in the dieting process.

We have learned, in previous chapters, how depressed and gloomy states of mind can increase the appetite and how a sense of joy and fulfillment makes dieting so much easier. In academic centers around the world, the revolutionary new study of neurochemistry has shown that those states of mind are not merely psychological. Not only does mood always have a chemical component, but that chemical component can actually be measured in a laboratory.

Dazzling as these discoveries have been, the field of neurochemistry is still in its infancy. Some findings are implied by the data collected thus far and some have been proved beyond doubt.

I have examined this fascinating data very carefully, and in my opinion there is a remarkable correlation between what they describe regarding the relationship of food and mood and what I have observed in my own clinical practice.

It is quite clear to me that certain measurable chemical entities in the food we eat strongly affect our emotions. There is no question in my mind that they help to make us happy or sad, and therefore help or hinder our dieting progress. Yet, till now *they have never been taken into account in any diet plan.*

Admittedly, the process by which the brain uses the contents of these foods to accomplish its miraculous feats is complex. Before we embark on an investigation of this process, let me tell you why I regard these discoveries as a heretofore "missing link" in the dieting process.

The biochemical factor in the Southampton Diet is the third in the four-point program you read about in Chapters 1 and 2. Specifically, it is a specially balanced diet designed to make certain that the proper amino acids reach your brain. The very same scientific investigations that have led to the dramatic changes in psychiatry have also revealed the powerful effects of these amino acids in the brain.

Certain amino acids can, when properly organized in a well-balanced nutritional meal plan, promote a stress-free diet. And though many diets claim to be stress-free, none, to my knowledge, has ever provided the ingredients that promote it. What *I* mean by a stress-free diet is one that will allow you to lose weight and at the same time not become excessively fatigued, unmotivated or irritable, hyper, manic or uncomfortable. I am thoroughly convinced that amino acids are the ingredients that have been overlooked by all other diets in the past, and that taking them into account and utilizing them properly not only makes sense in terms of the elimination of stress but also creates a qualitatively improved nutritional diet.

Understanding amino acids will shed light on their role in the dieting process.

Actually, these chemical entities are not acids at all. (You wouldn't suffer a burn by spilling one on your arm.) Amino acids are chemical agents contained in protein— sometimes called "the building blocks" of protein. They are molecular structures containing carbon, nitrogen and oxygen plus a certain R factor which influences the form and shape of each one of the twenty-two amino acids in the same way a gene affects the color of our eyes.

The chemical formula for an amino acid is as follows:

$$R - \overset{\displaystyle \overset{NH_2}{|}}{\underset{\displaystyle \underset{H}{|}}{C}} - C \overset{\displaystyle \nearrow O}{\underset{\displaystyle \searrow CH}{}}$$

What is important for us here is that R at the left. It is this factor which distinguishes one amino acid from another and, therefore, this factor which is important in relation to the brain and its control of the mind.

The new scientific evidence suggests the following:

Certain amino acids, each one of which has a different form dictated by that R factor, are capable of affecting our moods in different ways. To achieve true stress-free dieting, therefore, it is necessary to get the right amino acids into the body so they can help to produce the desired mood.

I will identify those amino acids later in this chapter. What is important to note at the moment is that they are in part— but not completely—contained in the food we eat.

As I mentioned earlier, the human body contains at least twenty-two amino acids. Of these, over half are generally described as "nonessential." These nonessential amino acids are produced within our bodies (though even these can be supplemented by food). The second, smaller group is called "essential," so named because we *must* supply them to our bodies through food. Both groups are of major concern in the Southampton Diet. For the first time in any diet plan, amino acids are carefully balanced throughout the meals so you will always consume exactly what you need. Nutritionally, this is extremely important. If an imbalance occurs or if some are actually missing altogether, our protein production is impaired, inhibited, even stopped. When that happens, our bodies deteriorate and we fall victim to disease.

But the nutritional value of amino acids is not the reason why I regard them as the missing link. I am vitally interested in amino acids because of the new discoveries about how they affect our moods and, therefore, our ability to diet comfortably.

Recent studies have shown that amino acids, once inside our bodies, change into what are called *neurotransmitters*. Neurotransmitters are, essentially, messengers to the brain. They can bring the brain either positive or negative information. Current scientific evidence indicates that often, by bringing positive information, they elevate our mood, and by bringing negative information they produce gloom or depression.

These neurotransmitters perform this function by flipping back and forth between one brain cell and another.

(Mental and mood alterations can actually be measured by the level of activity of various transmitter families.) In this process, the neurotransmitters often compete with one another to deliver their messages.

Our aim, of course, is to swell the forces of the positive neurotransmitters so that more of their messages will reach and enter the brain. The amino acid content of the Southampton Diet is designed to accomplish exactly that. It does this by including in every meal the amino acids that are known to produce positive neurotransmitters.

But there is another consideration. Both positive and negative neurotransmitters race to the brain by means of a variety of vehicles. We must also be concerned, therefore, with supplying the positive neurotransmitters with the vehicles that will get them to the brain in the fastest possible manner. In other words, since only a limited number of neurotransmitters can enter the brain at one time, we not only must increase their numbers but we must also provide them with proper transportation.

Like the neurotransmitters themselves, these various means of transportation can also be supplied by the nutrients in our diet. The Southampton Diet, therefore, provides a special orchestration of these nutrients to supply both the positive neurotransmitters and the vehicles they need to accomplish their work.

The following are examples of neurotransmitters formed from amino acids.

Probably the most important of the amino acids recently under examination is the one known as *tryptophan*. This is the amino acid that produces a positive neurotransmitter called *serotonin*. Studies at MIT* have shown that if the

* John H. Growdon, "Neurotransmitter precursors in the diet; Their use in the treatment of brain disease," in Nutrition and the Brain Series, vol. 3: *Disorders of Eating and Nutrients in Treatment of Brain Diseases*, eds. R. J. and J. J. Wurtman (New York: Raven Press, 1979), pp. 117–182.

level of serotonin in the brain falls too low, a person may experience depression, insomnia and unusually aggressive behavior.

One way to replenish serotonin in the brain is by ingesting the amino acid tryptophan. Medical research has revealed that tryptophan taken by mouth can both lift your spirits and help you sleep better. This miraculous amino acid accomplishes what appears to be such widely varied tasks by attacking that area of depression in which sleep patterns are disturbed. Unlike sleeping pills which, if taken regularly, will fragment sleep and lead to hangover and increased irritability once the pills are stopped, tryptophan stimulates the slow wave of sleep that is so important for both body repair and the calm, positive state of mind we have learned is the basis of stress-free dieting.

Still another example of an amino acid that affects our moods is *tyrosine*.

Like tryptophan, tyrosine is also used in the body to create neurotransmitters. In fact, tyrosine is a precursor of *two* of these busy brain messengers—dopamine and norepinephrine. (Dopamine is well known for its remarkable powers in the treatment of Parkinson's disease.)

The amino acid tyrosine has been used successfully to treat depression. In a recent study at Harvard University,* experimenters withdrew six depressed patients from the antidepressant medication they had been receiving. Three of them were given tyrosine several times a day and three were given placebo pills. All three tyrosine takers showed marked reduction of depression while the other three had to return to their original medication.

These and other studies have demonstrated most clearly that the ability of brain nerve cells to make and release

* "Neurotransmitter Precursors for the Treatment of Depression," A. J. Gelenberg, C. J. Gipson, and J. D. Wojcik; accepted for publication by *Psychopharmacology Bulletin*, 1982.

certain neurotransmitters depends directly on the concentration of amino acids in the blood.

What is even more remarkable is a further discovery: The level of those amino acids in the *most recent meal* that was eaten is the key. That is, the response in the brain could be measured almost immediately!

The series of experiments at MIT, which you read about earlier, showed how the brain messenger serotonin coordinates with the level of tryptophan in the blood. Furthermore, the experiments went on to prove, the tryptophan level fluctuated during the day in response to meals.

Amino acids, as we've said, are the building blocks of protein. Obviously, if you embark on a diet that supplies lots of carbohydrates and very little protein, you aren't going to supply your body with the proper amino acids. The Southampton Diet has carefully scheduled the proper proteinous foods that will provide you with exactly the amino acids you need. But, as I said before, eating lots of protein in all the right foods will not guarantee a happy mood at all times.

Certain foods that contain these amino acids as well as other nutrients are indeed very important to your mood. You will find them listed and explained in the next chapter.

But what is even more important is getting those amino acids and the neurotransmitters they produce to do the very best work they can. Again, the Southampton Diet accomplishes this by a very special balance of foods designed to help (that is, supply the vehicles for) those neurotransmitters.

This balance includes, for example, a certain small daily intake of *carbohydrates*. Carbohydrates, it has been found, are the vehicles that help the amino acid tryptophan increase its level in the bloodstream.

The Southampton Diet also includes a substantial portion of *B vitamins* which help the brain messenger serotonin.

Most depressed people lack B_3, B_6 and B_{12} in their diets. A deficiency of vitamin B_{12} often leads to mood changes, including depression, confusion and poor memory among the elderly. Those on strict vegetarian diets may also suffer a B_{12} deficiency because the vitamin is not found in plant life. A lack of vitamin B_1, or thiamine, may also lead to depression, according to two studies recently published by the federal government.* The most prominent behavioral effects of a diet depleted of vitamin B_1 are lethargy and fatigue. After eating a diet containing the recommended amount of vitamin B_1, the subjects' behavior returned to normal. In the second study, marginal deficiencies of B_2 (riboflavin) and vitamin C also led to depression.

Folic acid and vitamin C are also two important ingredients in the Southampton Diet. In combination, they play a role in the formation of dopamine.

Furthermore, although amino acids and their products, the neurotransmitters, play the central role in the Southampton Diet, I have also made certain that every nutritional need of the human body is met. Unlike amino acids, most of these nutrients have not—or not *yet*—been linked to the production of neurotransmitters, but scientific studies *have* shown their relationship to mood.

You will find a description of all of these nutrients, along with the foods that contain them, in the next chapter. Included in this list are all those foods that contain the missing link—the amino acids that play such a remarkable role in the creation of neurotransmitters.

Discovering the role played by the chemical properties

* Myron Brin, "Example of Behavioral Changes in Marginal Vitamin Deficiency in the Rat and Man" (Proceedings of International Nutrition Conference, "Behavioral Effects of Energy and Protein Deficits"), NIH Publication no. 79-1906 (August 1979), pp. 272–277.

in food was one of the most important steps in my own 210-pound weight loss. As I mentioned earlier, I had suspected that such a connection existed when I was in medical school. I had found, for example, that a certain amount of milk made my dieting easier, while chocolate created an emotional letdown that made dieting more difficult.

It was only after several years and much examination of the experimental work in psychochemistry that I came to the conclusion that the chemical ingredients in both of those foods were actually *producing* these emotional effects.

I have, in creating the Southampton Diet, eliminated any food that could produce negative neurotransmitters, and I have included every food now known to elevate mood.

Although, as I said, the study of psychochemistry is still in its infancy, I see the results of this special chemical balance every day in my practice. Once my patients begin the Southampton Diet, their initial depression soon lifts. They are invariably more cheerful and less subject to mood swings. Although it may seem surprising that the choice of food should influence such an important process as the creation of neurotransmitters and subsequent mood changes, I see the evidence of it daily in my office. Dieting, for the overwhelming number of my patients, is more pleasant and successful than any of them imagined was possible.

I am certain you, too, will find, when you proceed on the Southampton Diet, that while you are losing weight, you will feel neither hungry nor depressed. Your spirits will lift as your appetite falls.

5

HAPPY FOODS, SAD FOODS

THIS CHAPTER WILL PROVIDE YOU with a list of the foods that can influence mood. It will also describe some of the biochemical properties of these foods and how they affect your emotions.

As we begin listing these "happy" and "sad" foods, however, we must bear in mind what we learned in the last chapter: For most of the happy foods to take their full effect, they must be ingested along with certain foods. This careful balance is what you will be eating on the Southampton Diet. You will find that the diet contains many meals which provide the amino acid tryptophan simultaneously with carbohydrates to produce the combined effect of happy food.

Scientific studies have proved that tryptophan is most effective in elevating moods when up to six grams are ingested each day. Taking more is not as effective. The Southampton Diet provides about one gram a day of tryptophan with, of course, an appropriate amount of carbohydrates to get the tryptophan into the brain to do its antidepressant work. Tryptophan is found in a wide range of foods, among them turkey, chicken and cottage cheese.

As I have noted earlier, most of us who are overweight are experiencing at the same time a certain minor level of depression. We may not be *clinically* depressed, just feeling "down" simply *because* we are overweight. Adding happy foods that provide the amino acid tyrosine helps us to get through that difficult time by actually making us feel good biochemically. Tyrosine is present in red meats and milk and, in smaller amounts, in fruits and vegetables.

You will find that although red meats, organ meats and milk are often excluded from many other diets, eaten in small amounts and in the proper combinations, you will be able to enjoy them, feel good and still lose weight on the Southampton Diet.

One way to step up the production of the neurotransmitter serotonin and alleviate a depressed mood is to boost the levels of B vitamins in the diet. The happy foods that contain vitamin B_{12} include organ meats such as liver, kidney and heart, also fish, eggs, cheese and milk products. For B_6: whole grains, yeast, wheat germ, leafy green vegetables, and brown rice. Foods high in B_3 (also known as niacin) are organ meats, fish, yeast, and rice bran.

As we learned in Chapter 4, folic acid and vitamin C in combination play a role in the formation of the neurotransmitter dopamine. A deficiency in folic acid has been known to lead to feelings of depression and confusion. Since supplementing a diet with folic acid can counter depression, foods rich in this nutrient are also prescribed on the Southampton Diet. These happy foods that contain folic acid are green leafy vegetables, meats, whole grains, yeast, oysters, salmon and milk. I recommend combining folic acid foods with foods containing vitamin C, such as citrus fruits, strawberries, broccoli, tomatoes and green peppers.

Federal studies linking vitamin B_1 and B_2 with mood changes were cited in the last chapter. These vitamins are present in whole grains, yeast, organ meats and leafy vegetables. You will find many of these vitamin-rich foods on the Southampton Diet.

Deficiencies of iron, potassium and magnesium in the blood can produce chronic fatigue. For high energy and a "spunky" feeling throughout the day, the Southampton Diet includes organ meats, eggs, fish, poultry, green leafy vegetables for *potassium*, and fish, whole grains, dark green vegetables and milk for *magnesium*.

You will find all these on my list of happy foods.

Among the sad foods (or the ingredients in sad foods) is, first and foremost, sugar. Most of us have felt that rush just after eating a candy bar, as blood-sugar levels rise. And then the letdown as the sweet stuff becomes fully metabolized. Perhaps a mild depression may even set in.

Low blood-sugar levels can lead to a condition called hypoglycemia and feelings of depression and irritability. Insulin, as you may know, is a substance which controls the level of glucose (sugar) in your blood. If insulin production is impaired, your blood-sugar level will suffer and your moods will fluctuate. Eating a balanced diet will keep your blood-sugar level stable without the roller-coaster ride of moods that comes from satisfying a sweet tooth.

Another, and most important, way to avoid the ups and downs of the so-called sugar blues is to stretch out your food intake over the day. The Southampton Diet, with a midday snack and dessert eaten two hours after dinner, provides you with small surges of insulin so that you can feel happy throughout the day as you are dieting. In short, you will maintain a steady insulin level.

Your body's production of insulin is also helpful in another way. Insulin, it has been discovered, increases the level of the amino acid tryptophan. It does this by causing a rapid reduction in other competing amino acids. When the level of these competing amino acids, which include leucine, isoleucine and phenylalanine, drops, tryptophan can make faster headway into the brain.

Your intake of sugar should be controlled for another reason. When you eat sweets, you steal vitamins from their limited stores in your cells. This may lead to vitamin B depletion, which, as we mentioned, can reduce your efficiency and depress your mood.

Avoiding the sugar blues is only one reason why the Southampton Diet provides snacks to be spaced out over the day. The other reason is that eating small amounts of food more often requires the body to expend more energy, and therefore more calories, than if you gorge yourself at one or two sittings. Some diets actually recommend that you have one big meal a day. This may be all right for your dog, but I don't advocate a dog's diet for you. The more energy you expend, the more calories you will burn up and the more weight you will subsequently lose. It's as simple as that.

Chocolate is another food on the sad list. It contains a substance that creates a negative neurotransmitter, phenylalanine, and is a sad food when eaten regularly and in large amounts, as many overweight people do. There is a good deal of evidence to suggest that a craving for chocolate represents a physical substitution for emotional needs: most often for love, affection, or sex. (A reversal of that craving will be discussed in Chapter 6.)

Certain high-fat foods tend to make you feel sleepy and tired. Therefore, emulsifiers like *lecithin*, which hold fats together and allow them to mix well, are on the sad side of the ledger. Lowering the levels of lecithin in your diet may help to promote a more energetic lifestyle. On the sad-foods list, therefore, are all fatty foods and marbled meats.

Another drawback to lecithin is that it contains a substance called *choline*. A number of researchers have noted that high doses of choline appear to exacerbate depression.

73

One of the side effects of treating patients with the disease tardive dyskinesia (involuntary facial movements) appears to be a withdrawal and depression, apparently related to choline intake. A by-product of choline, acetylcholine, docs block the action of dopamine, which, you will remember, may cause depression if the brain has a low level of this neurotransmitter. Foods containing choline are on the list of sad foods. They include mayonnaise, all fatty foods and marbled meats.

Using seasonings that contain monosodium glutamate (MSG) is not recommended. MSG can cause drowsiness and headache, dizziness and other unpleasant feelings. It has been associated with depression as well. Most people who have reactions to MSG in foods fully recover in a few minutes or hours. But the glutamate releases sugar stores from the liver and can make glucose unavailable when it's needed later.

And then there is lobster. Unfortunately, this delicious luxury contains a high concentration of GABA, gamma aminobutyric acid, an inhibitory neurotransmitter of the brain. Increased levels of GABA can lead to a very logy and lethargic lifestyle. Since lethargy is the exact opposite of the happy, productive manner in which my patients wish to live, lobster is not included on the Southampton Diet.

Similarly, large amounts of lentils and chick-peas will act as depressants and inhibit the thyroid gland. You will find these foods as well on the sad side of the ledger.

HAPPY FOODS

Milk Turkey Chicken Unripened Cheese Beef Bananas Pineapple Yogurt	Contain Tryptophan
Lean Red Meat: beef, plus game meats, but excluding pork Organ Meats: liver, kidney, heart	Contain Tyrosine
Fish Eggs (contain vitamin B) Whole Grains Yeast Wheat Germ Green Leafy Vegetables Brown Rice Rice Bran (shell of rice)	Contain B Vitamins and Folic Acid
Oranges Grapefruit Lemons or Limes Strawberries Broccoli Green Peppers Spinach Brussels Sprouts Cantaloupe	Contain Vitamin C

75

SAD FOODS

Sugar
Mayonnaise } **Produce Sugar Blues**
Fatty Foods

Marbled Meats } **Contain Choline**

Chocolate } **Contains Phenylalanine**

Aged Cheese
Pickled Herring
Chianti
Sour Cream } **Contain Tyramine, a Competitor of Tyrosine**
Beer
Ripe Avocados
Aged Beef

Food with MSG } **Associated with Depression**

Lobster } **Contains GABA**

Lentils
Chick-peas } **Inhibit Thyroid**

76

6

SEX AND YOUR WEIGHT

WE HAVE ALL SEEN—and perhaps you have re-
marked on this phenomenon yourself—how well an acquaintance looks when she or he has "fallen in love."
Sometimes we may meet this friend for the first time after
a recent marriage or, now that society's sexual standards
have changed, since she or he has moved in with a new
lover.

"You look marvelous," we say to this blooming creature
and, more often than not, "Have you lost weight?"

Chances are the answer to that question is "Yes."

As we have learned in previous chapters, happiness tends
to decrease our appetites and our blissful friend has undoubtedly responded to that emotional impetus as well.

But something else may be happening to our friend, too.
An increase in sexual activity, in and of itself, also actually
helps us to lose weight. Sex accomplishes this supportive
feat in two ways, the first psychological, and the second
physical.

As we learned in Chapter 3, overeating often creates a
Fat Shield that separates us from the rest of the world.
Usually, we are separating ourselves from something

we very much desire, but are too timid to ask or negotiate for.

Another way to describe this psychological maneuver, the term psychoanalysts most often use, is *sublimation*.

Sublimation involves the substitution of a secondary desire for a primary one. When we overeat, as distinguished from eating because we're hungry, we are frequently replacing a primary desire for sex or affection with a secondary desire for the oral gratification of eating.

This is not surprising when we consider the close similarity between the sensual stimulation of food and that of sex. For one thing, both involve the sensitive oral zone. For another, as infants, our earliest experience combined both nourishment and sensual pleasure as we suckled at the breast. Even adults, I suspect, enjoy their most satisfying sexual encounters when their subconscious returns to the sensual memory state in which they are feeding at their mother's breast.

Most of us who are afflicted with weight problems can recall at least one incident in our lives when we found ourselves reaching for food when our desire for intimate contact with another person was frustrated. Those of us with a sweet tooth can probably recall a myriad of such incidents.

The substitution of food for intimacy has been quite well documented in the case of sweets—chocolate in particular. Chocolate, we have found, can create emotional sensations quite similar to those we feel when we are in love. Medical research has pinpointed a certain chemical activity in our brain that occurs during a period of what we might call infatuation or early courtship. This chemical activity produces an emotional high almost exactly like that produced by eating chocolate. (We have even identified the activating substance in chocolate. This is the chemical entity known as phenylethylamine, and you will find it high on the list of sad foods.)

Since the psychic response to eating chocolate and falling in love are so similar, it is only logical to assume that we might easily be substituting a *secondary* desire for sweet food for the *primary* need for physical or romantic intimacy.

And if, in fact, we *do* find ourselves filling a wish for closeness through the self-punishing route of ingesting sweets, chocolate or other fattening caloric intake, what should we do about it? The answer is really just as simple as the original exchange itself. There is no reason that I know of why we can't reverse the process and substitute sexual intimacy for overeating.

I will recommend several methods of accomplishing this later in this chapter, but before I do, let's take a look at how this food/sex reversal worked for two of my patients.

Margery was one of those patients. She was a pretty, round-faced, twenty-three-year-old blonde, the wife of the owner of a chic and popular restaurant in Southampton. She came to my office six months after the birth of her first child, weighing about thirty pounds more than she wanted to weigh.

During the course of our first interview, it became obvious that the new baby was the center of Margery's life. She not only took great delight in the child but followed every single prescription for caring for it that she had ever read in a child-care book or heard from friends or relatives.

Needless to say, all these dos and don'ts of child-rearing took up most of Margery's attention. There was very little left for anything or anyone else, including her husband.

Every day, Margery told me, she would wheel the baby in her carriage along the main street of Southampton, stopping in the pastry and candy shops for snacks. Every night, she would fall into bed exhausted. By the time her husband returned home from his restaurant, she was sound asleep.

When I inquired about her sex life, Margery's blue eyes opened wide in surprise.

"I don't know," she replied. "I guess I haven't thought much about it since the baby was born." She had not, she continued, made love with her husband for several months. Apparently, Margery had assumed from all her reading that her new role in life was to spend all her time caring for her child.

"I'd hardly call this a balanced existence," I suggested. Margery agreed. Furthermore, she admitted, her husband had been growing increasingly snappish and distant in the past few months, and this worried her.

As Margery began the Southampton Diet, I recommended that she make an attempt to resume some sort of sexual activity with her husband, even if it was only once or twice a week. Not only was this important to her marriage and to the parental environment her baby required, but I suspected that the absence of sex may have been contributing to her weight gain as well. The baby, I assured Margery, would not suffer if she saved some of her energy for her husband and made herself more available to him sexually.

When Margery returned for her appointment the next week, she had lost ten of her thirty-pound weight gain. But even more noticeable was the rosy glow of her cheeks. Her face had lost some of its roundness and I could hardly avoid remarking to her, as to that anonymous acquaintance we spoke of earlier, "You look marvelous!"

Resuming her sex life was not only important to Margery's marriage, but the sensual gratification she received from it actually replaced what had been a driving desire for pastries and candy. Since that desire had literally melted away, "the rest," she announced, "would be easy."

And indeed it was. It wasn't long before Margery was stopping in at her husband's restaurant in the evening, her figure at least as stunning as it had been before the baby was born.

Clearly, Margery had accomplished the food/sex reversal. She had substituted sexual intimacy for food instead of —as she had been doing before—the other way around.

But there is yet another way in which sex functions to help us lose weight; that is, through its excellent value as exercise and the actual burning of calories it provides. Because sexual activity is usually—and rightfully—closely linked to our emotional lives, we seldom think of it simply as exercise. But the fact of the matter is that healthy, active sex *does* burn calories. Though it's difficult to assign an exact caloric expenditure rate to the average act of sexual intercourse (difficult even to determine what is *average* sexual intercourse!), we do know that added calories are burned during coitus. A fair estimate is that the body uses up about 200 calories during any period of physical intimacy that culminates in orgasm.

There is certainly no question that sex requires *some* increased energy expenditure. One indication alone—the pulse rate of a sexually aroused human being—*has* been measured and found to be as high as 150 beats per minute, a major increase from the normal 70 beats per minute.

The value of sex as exercise was pointed out to me by an acquaintance who later became a patient of mine. She was (and is) one of the most celebrated beauties in New York —we'll call her Judith—and she was very much in love with her husband, Arthur, a television executive.

Judith was in her middle forties when I first saw her at a gala dinner given by mutual friends. She was the center of attention and amused us all with her lighthearted response to compliments. She had kept her youth and lovely figure, she joked, through frequent exercise—in bed!

I met Judith again several years later when, to my surprise, she entered my office as a patient. She had gained twenty pounds and though, to my eyes, she was still very lovely, she insisted that she must lose the added weight or, she said with a wry laugh, "invest in a whole new wardrobe!"

During the course of the interview, I reminded this charming woman of the dinner party we had attended and of her amusing remarks on the subject of sex as exercise. To my surprise, she did not respond in her usual witty manner, but answered very soberly that the matter of sex was no longer a joke. Then she explained.

Six months earlier Arthur had suffered a mild stroke. He was diagnosed as hypertensive; that is, he had high blood pressure. Judith was terrified of resuming what had truly been their active sex life because she feared precipitating another stroke. Yet she had never expressed this fear to Arthur and had simply avoided all sexual encounters with him.

I immediately suggested to Judith that she was mistaken to assume that her love for Arthur was best expressed by remaining silent about something that had once been such a vital part of their lives.

"Perhaps," I said, "if you explained this sudden reticence, Arthur would actually feel better about it." Furthermore, I added, it might be a good idea for Arthur to take the problem directly to his neurologist.

Judith quickly agreed to this plan. Like most partners in a finely tuned relationship, she had been uncomfortable hiding her feelings from her husband.

Judith did not wait for her next appointment to fill me in on the encouraging results. She telephoned two days later. Arthur's physician had thoroughly reassured both of them. Sex was certainly *not* contraindicated for Arthur and would pose no danger to his neurological condition. Judith's happy, healthy "exercise" was restored to her and, by sticking with the diet, she brought her weight down rapidly.

Judith agreed—as did Margery—that the resumption of an active sex life was an enormous help in losing weight.

Now, I grant you that in both of these cases the solution to an atrophied sex life was relatively easy. Unlike many overweight people, both of these women had potential partners who were convenient and willing.

It is indeed a bit more difficult for those of us who are single.

But another side of this argument must also be considered: Margery and Judith were both carrying between twenty to thirty pounds of extra weight when they approached their husbands with sexual overtures. These two women were not immune to the feelings that most of us suffer from when we are overweight. We all know what that prevalent emotion (and our biggest hurdle) is. It is a sense of embarrassment about our bodies.

This sense of embarrassment—or shame—is certainly understandable in the light of all we have learned about the Fat Shield.

Our Fat Shields, you may remember, were originally created by our desire to avoid dealing with certain personal relationships. Among those relationships are, of course, the sexual ones. Our sense of embarrassment thus serves an unconscious and self-defeating purpose—avoidance of the very experiences we most desire.

Furthermore, as we have learned, the Fat Shield is self-perpetuating. As we isolate ourselves, we become depressed; as we become depressed, we tend to eat more.

You have seen how this self-defeating cycle is broken the moment we begin the Southampton Diet. Sexual activity battles the cycle on another front, by directly attacking the isolation and consequent depression.

Now, I am not going to insist that you are wrong if, being an overweight person, you see yourself as less sought-after as a sexual partner than your slimmer acquaintances. In today's society, the chances are that this perception is fairly accurate. As I have observed every day on the beaches and discotheques of Southampton, the quality of thinness has an influence on success in most areas of life, including that of attracting sexual partners. Most of these powerful people —whether their names are known to the public or whether their influence is felt behind the scenes—are slim. This factor, plus the good health that accompanies a slender body, is the reason you intend to lose all that unwanted weight.

It is also true, however, that you can enjoy the pleasures of sex before you have reached your ultimate weight goal. The sense of shame or embarrassment you may feel because your body is not yet as slender as it will be is unnecessary and self-defeating.

The truth is that there is nothing inherently shameful in being overweight. In fact, during certain historical periods, a plump body was considered most desirable and attractive. What is important for you, as for most of my patients, to realize is that increased sexual activity is simply another means by which you intend to achieve your ultimate goal —to be "Southampton thin."

As I have said, caring for yourself is the basic principle of the Southampton Diet program.

What I am suggesting here is just another facet of caring for yourself. I am suggesting that you give yourself the gift of sensuous and pleasurable sexual encounters.

By sensuous and pleasurable sexual encounters I do not mean: 1) competitive performances in which each party displays his or her body for judgment, *or* 2) sexual gymnastics contests, *or* 3) single-minded sexual marathons aimed solely at orgasm.

I mean intimate relationships in which the senses of a healthy mind and body are engaged. This includes the senses of touching and being touched, of hearing and being heard; it includes the senses of smell and taste. And it involves using these senses to explore all areas of your partner's body as well as enjoying your partner's exploration of your own body. It means receiving pleasure through giving it, and vice versa.

According to this description, sensuous and pleasurable sexual encounters cannot be in any way off limits for an overweight person.

Furthermore, though there are no definitive studies to date on this matter, it is my opinion that people who tend toward weight problems also tend to be more adept at employing their senses, and perhaps even more developed sensually than others. The chances are, then, that they are more likely to enjoy giving and receiving sensual pleasure.

A sensitivity to one's senses is the quality which—above all else—creates the most sublime and exciting sexual relationships. If you have been reticent about sex because of an unnecessary and self-defeating sense of embarrassment, you have been depriving *yourself* of your sensual gifts, and others as well.

Be assured that increasing your sexual activity will aid you in becoming Southampton thin. Toward that goal— and in the interest of attracting a sexual partner—I suggest the following:

The simplest way to achieve that awareness is through the exploration of your own body. To begin with, you should relegate any sense of embarrassment to the ash heap of useless prejudice where it belongs and freely examine your own erogenous zones, those parts of your body that are most responsive to all those senses mentioned above—especially, in this case, the sense of touch. You should give full attention and freedom to yourself as a sensuous human being and ascertain your personal areas of arousal and your favorite method of stimulation.

This erotic self-exploration is, as I'm sure you know, usually described as masturbation, and you may be wondering if I am recommending masturbation as a method of weight loss.

In fact, under certain circumstances, I *do* recommend it, most specifically when there are no partners available (which is highly unlikely unless the patient happens to be marooned on an ice floe in Alaska). Primarily, however, I suggest masturbation merely as a step toward realizing one's own full interpersonal sexual potential.

Learning about your own sensuality through self-exploration is the best method I know to provide the confidence you need to approach potential sexual partners. Your body's response to your own touch is your clue to how the bodies of others will respond. When you have satisfied yourself, you will be better able to satisfy others. And this, after all, is what most potential partners are seeking.

My second recommendation for a more active sex life is simply this: During your weight-loss period, apply extra effort in the area of socialization. Go out more often—to parties, meetings, hotels, theater, art or civic groups; join a club or political organization—anything and anywhere that one might expect to meet new friends and/or potential partners. If you encounter someone you have reason to think might be of interest to you, approach him or her and initiate a conversation. (A compliment is usually a pleasant introduction, particularly when it's sincere.) Be prepared for the fact that not every person you approach will accept your offer. In the long run, however, your initiative is bound to be rewarded.

I have found in my experience with so many patients—even among those who are so obviously attractive and successful—that loneliness is one of the most common and painful afflictions of our time. Relationships in our mobile society shift constantly, and most people are looking and hoping for exactly what your extra effort is designed to achieve—a satisfying personal intimacy.

What is required is only a comparatively minor degree of effort. The sexual revolution has created a vast pool of potential participants who would not have been available twenty years ago. This means that the added time and energy you must expend in seeking out a relationship is probably the same or even less than your slender competitor would have applied twenty years ago!

As you begin on the Southampton Diet, you should add reenergizing and revitalizing sexual pleasure to your new life-changing program. If you have a great deal of weight to lose, it may be helpful to know that the following coital positions are comfortable for the obese:

If the woman is obese:
• She lies on her side with the knee of her upper leg bent and drawn up toward her chest. The male kneels on the bed, placing one knee on either side of her lower, straight leg. His penis enters her vagina from the rear, at a slight angle.
• The female lies on her back on the bed. She bends her knees and opens her legs as wide as she can. This is a standard position. It is used in gynecological examinations because it provides the greatest exposure of the vagina and vulva.

If the man is obese:
• He lies on his back on the bed and the woman straddles his genital area, either on her knees or in a squatting position. She then inserts his penis into her vagina. Coital thrusts are, in this case, mainly the prerogative of the female, but the male can often participate by raising or lowering his hips.
• If, after assuming this position, the couple rolls to the side, the female can still regulate her movements.

If both partners are obese:
• The female kneels, lowering her chest toward the bed and

arching her back slightly. Her knees should be several inches apart. The male enters from the rear and can then rest on the female's buttocks during the thrust of sexual intercourse.

There are other positions, of course, and I assume you will be experimenting with many of them. Most of my patients have reported that their sexual imaginations expand as their waistlines diminish. They have found—as I'm sure you will—that sex becomes even more enjoyable as they lose weight, if only because slimmer bodies make for easier and deeper genital penetration.

You may have noticed, by the way, that though the Southampton Diet provides for frequent snacks, none are specified for late at night or postcoital. This is because the sexual gratification that will successfully substitute for food must be sensitive, erotic and *complete*. That pleasure is not obtained in a quick or mechanical manner. It is a long, sensuous process in which all phases, including foreplay, coitus and, most important, *afterplay* are essential.

Most of us realize that foreplay and coitus are vital parts of our enjoyment of sex. I consider afterplay equally important because, though a healthy, happy sex life is much to be desired in and of itself, the goal of this book is to assure your weight loss. Afterplay is directly connected to that goal because there is a common complaint in this regard that I have heard so often in my practice that I now have it framed and hanging on the wall of my office.

"But Dr. Berger," it reads, "I get so hungry after sex!"

My answer to that is usually quite direct.

"If you get hungry after sex, it's because you have forgotten something."

More often than not, people who have a desire for food following sexual intercourse have omitted a most important component of a satisfying sexual encounter. They have forgotten the afterplay—that period following coitus when lovers hold each other in their arms, adding caresses to the caresses that have brought them so much pleasure. This phase of lovemaking can bring the ultimate satisfaction of the sex act—the sense of truly being loved and wanted. It is the final fulfillment.

Obviously, if this period has been ignored, if you and your partner have drawn apart before it is completed, you are bound to feel deprived. This deprivation—not true hunger—is the reason you may, at that point, experience what you interpret as a need to eat something.

You will not find that "something" on the Southampton Diet. You will, I hope, have no need for it, because you will remember to pleasure both yourself and your partner with leisurely, prolonged afterplay.

You will also, I am sure, enjoy all the rewards of a newly expanded sex life: the sense of vitality, good health, self-esteem and last—but certainly not least—a rapid weight loss.

And if you're tempted at any time by a forbidden sweet, please remember to examine your own affectional life. You will find, I am certain, that increased sexual activity offers a much better, more life-sustaining and energizing solution, one that will aid the Southampton Diet in providing you with the program through which you will be thin and happy for the rest of your life.

7

HOW TO STAY ON THE SOUTHAMPTON DIET

THE PROBLEM OF OVERWEIGHT has proved to be one of the most stubborn in medical and psychiatric history. No simple miracle cure, no vaccine or antibiotic, has appeared on the horizon to immediately dismiss this painful issue from our homes and hospitals. Over the years, a human being's tendency to overweight has shown itself to be highly resistant to most forms of therapy.

I believe that the reason for this resistance is the complexity of the problem and, therefore, the great number of stimuli that can feed into and exacerbate it. As I've said before, this was the conclusion I reached in my own eventually successful attempt to engineer and maintain a 210-pound weight loss. Because of the problem's complexity, no *one* approach can address it satisfactorily. For a comprehensive attack one must draw from several disciplines. This is the reasoning behind the four-point system of the Southampton Diet. Each of these points addresses the problem of overweight on a different level.

You have read about three of these points in detail in previous chapters. The first is the diet itself, with its carefully orchestrated nutritional balance. The second point—the Fat Shield—allows you to understand the degree to which the accumulation of fat acts as self-punishment. The third is the mood/food connection, the biochemical balance of foods that provides the mood elevation necessary to keep you happy while you are dieting. And the fourth, which you will read more about here, is behavioral therapy.

As I have stated previously, I believe that behavioral therapy is far more effective in the treatment of overweight than traditional psychotherapeutic approaches. I have used behavioral techniques myself, on my own weight-loss *and* maintenance regime, and they have provided essential tools for most of my patients.

Current behavioral therapy's theoretical roots lie in the original work done by B. F. Skinner and J. B. Watson who, in turn, drew on the theories of the Russian physiologist Ivan Petrovich Pavlov. A great deal of this work focused on human response to external or internal stimuli—i.e., cues. Later behavioral research, building on this base, expanded into more particular and specific areas, among them an examination of the operation of the stimulus-response dynamic in the area of everyday patterns of nutritional sustenance—i.e., how people eat.

Several fairly solid conclusions were reached through this research. Among them, for example, is the observation that overweight people react more strongly to the external stimuli of food than do those who do not have an overweight problem.

What this means, in everyday terms, is that people who tend to overeat do so when they see or smell attractive food, rather than when they are hungry. Those who do not have weight problems, on the other hand, tend to eat primarily when they are hungry (an internal stimulus) and are seldom tempted by external visual or olfactory cues.

A variety of studies has born out this thesis. Several of them found that thin members of a random group of people eat less if they had eaten an hour or so earlier, more if a longer time period had occurred between meals. Heavier people, on the other hand, were found to eat more if the food was attractively prepared. If the food was not appealing either to view or taste, however, those who were overweight tended to dismiss it, even if an extended time period had elapsed since their last meal and it could be logically concluded that they were hungry.

This particular conclusion is one that I have validated to my own satisfaction both by careful questioning of my patients and by observing people at gatherings where they are exposed to large amounts of attractive food. And most of us who must battle overweight can recognize the accuracy of these observations in ourselves. Certainly, I found this phenomenon to be true during my years in medical school and internship when I was struggling to lose so much weight. Often many hours would go by—while I was on duty in the hospital, busy and vitally interested in the patients under my care—and I would feel no need for food, no awareness of hunger. After my shift, I generally stopped at the hospital cafeteria for a meal (which was dull but sufficient) and then returned to my room. There, inevitably—at least in the early days of my dieting—I would automatically open my refrigerator to view my stock of what I now realize were stimuli—salamis, Cokes, cakes, et cetera. What a surge of "hunger" I experienced then, even though I had eaten less than an hour earlier!

Of course, this desire to eat was not really hunger at all, but, at least in part, the typical overeater's response to food cues. (The other parts of my response were the result of inadequacies in my early diet program.)

It was many years before I was able to cull from behavioral research exactly those techniques that best answered my own problem in this area. You will find those techniques I found most effective listed in this chapter, along with several others that have proved valuable to my patients. Not *all* of these procedures will be appropriate for you. It is important to identify your own particular response patterns first. Then you can, as I did myself and as each of my patients does, apply the special technique that exactly answers your needs.

Identifying your own stimulus-response pattern is best achieved by means of illustration. The following, therefore, is a list of patient examples that I find best illuminate the most typical—and universal—patterns of overeating.

Myra, age thirty-six, producer of television documentaries and mother of three children, twelve pounds overweight:

Myra had no difficulty at all staying on the Southampton Diet during the day. In the evenings, however, when she was preparing meals for her husband and children, she was often tempted to do more than simply *taste* her own cooking. Her kitchen, she reported, was a large, comfortable place; the children often did their homework there and, not coincidentally, spent time with their mother there. During those hours, Myra said, "temptation was everywhere."

I have a special sympathy for those of you who, like Myra, are responsible for preparing meals. You are almost *trapped* in the kitchen area by the cues that, we have learned, usually trigger overeating. Any one of the following techniques will ease the problem; using all of them will totally release you from the entrapment:

1. Cook all the food at the same time, thus shortening the time period spent in the kitchen.

2. After dinner, be certain that someone other than yourself clears the table and cleans the kitchen—i.e., do not return there.

3. Remove all electronic or other socialization equipment from the kitchen. This might include a telephone or television, or, as in Myra's case, the table on which the children wrote their homework. The aim here is to change the kitchen environment from an area of socialization to one of food preparation only. (Myra found that by shortening her cooking period, she was able to spend time with the children in another room of the house. She also used the following technique on alternate days.)

4. Assign someone else to prepare meals. This is possible more often than you may think. Many of my patients report that, as their spouses and children realize the seriousness and obvious success rate of the Southampton Diet, they are more willing—even highly interested in—cooperating on the project.

William, forty-two years old. Museum curator and painter; eight pounds overweight:

Bill was particularly susceptible to the sight of food. Both his vocation and avocation were highly oriented toward the visual aspects of life. Furthermore, he worked at home a good deal and was constantly fighting the desire to pop into his mouth a sugary almond or a truffle from one of the lovely bowls he kept on small tables. "But one can't," Bill complained, "divest one's home of all forms of sustenance."

Of course that's true. Yet, if you are usually responsive to the sight of food, that "sustenance" should not extend to heaping bowls of confections widely distributed where you are likely to see them often.

Techniques that effectively circumvent the problem of high visual sensitivity are:

1. Remove all high-caloric foods from open containers and store them on the highest, most inaccessible shelf.

2. Buy and store foods in opaque containers.

3. Rearrange your refrigerator so that any food that is not prescribed on the Southampton Diet is hidden from sight, or at least *first* sight. If you have reached the maintenance level of the diet, proceed similarly.

Elizabeth, fifty years old, novelist, weight loss twenty pounds, beginning maintenance diet:

Elizabeth's difficulty was what is often described as "response to situational stimuli." Before she began the Southampton Diet, she tended to snack, and thus overeat, when she was working. (Similar situations that evoke this response are watching television, attending sports events, reading, talking on the phone.)

The regimen of the Southampton Diet changed Elizabeth's eating patterns quite radically, but since snacks are provided on the diet, she had continued to eat them during the time periods she spent at the typewriter. Although Elizabeth lost twenty pounds quite easily on the diet, she feared, as she began the more relaxed maintenance regimen, that she might return to the heavy snacking that had been, in part, the cause of her weight gain.

The technique I prescribed for Elizabeth (and one I use myself to maintain my own weight) is as follows:

Designate one area (and one area alone) of your home in which *all* food is consumed. (In my case, it is the dining-room table.) If, while you are reading, watching television, or whatever your own situational stimulus might be, you feel a desire to eat, leave the book or television set and go to the designated eating area to consume the food.

This simple act is a powerful tool for breaking this particular response pattern. As an ancillary benefit, it forces an awareness of the degree to which the food you consume is actually the response to true desire on your part, rather than automatic, mindless eating.

Further support for this awareness can be achieved in a

wider environment than the home. This is accomplished by forbidding yourself to consume food while you are engaged in any activity (other than conversation with a dinner companion). Do not eat, for example, while you are walking along the street or even riding in the car. Your actual desire for the food in question will soon become apparent.

Beverly, twenty-six years old, pediatrician, five pounds overweight:

Beverly lost her five pounds within a week, but because she had, prior to this point, developed a pattern that is so common to overeaters, I have included her problem here.

This young physician had recently opened an office in Southampton. She was highly credentialed and had no reason to doubt that she would eventually have a busy practice. For the moment, however, her patients were few and she waited long hours between them. During these periods, Beverly was often bored and anxious and tended to nibble fruit and cheese from the office refrigerator.

Though it may be difficult to imagine boredom or anxiety as a stimulus, in the area of overeating, either or both are, in fact, the most pernicious. The problem they present, however, is one that lends itself to a relatively precise solution.

Few of my patients lead simple lives. Most are confronted with many demands and tasks they have to accomplish, as well as pleasures they wish to enjoy. The technique I suggest to them, and to you, if you recognize this boredom or anxiety/eating response in yourself, is as follows:

Make an ongoing list of activities you must accomplish or would enjoy carrying out. This list should have no boundaries. It should include everything from visiting a friend or cleaning a cupboard to balancing a checkbook, taking a leisurely bath or going to a local art gallery. (If the enjoyment level is high, all the better.)

Keep the list easily available. The moment you sense the onset of an anxious or boring waiting period, turn to it immediately. Choose one of the tasks or pleasures and begin to carry it out instantly. If you substitute this new response to the old stimuli several times, you will soon notice that the power of this situational stimulus will gradually dissipate. In time, the weakening effect will be such that eventually the entire pattern will undoubtedly vanish.

This technique is, essentially, a behavioral *replacement* method; that is, a different response (from your list) replaces the original (eating). Another very effective technique involves direct confrontation of the stimuli. For example:

Jane, thirty-nine years old, a popular Southampton hostess, weight loss thirteen pounds, beginning maintenance diet:

Jane was the daughter of great wealth and a somewhat moralistic upbringing. Although she was very much her own woman in most respects, she had, like most of us, a certain degree of unconscious residue remaining from earlier parental strictures. Within it was the far-from-uncommon guilt about leaving food on her plate that would then be discarded or, as she put it, "wasted, while others go hungry."

I'm sure I need not, at this point, launch into a discussion of the skewed view of reality this sort of reasoning presents, or of how, in fact, consuming all the food on one's plate in no way assists the "starving children in Asia," or whatever the current parental injunction. Instead, let's directly confront this inducement to overeating, as I did for Jane.

"Your new rule," I told her, "is exactly the opposite. It is: Always leave some food on your plate."

Jane was amused at this reversal, but agreed to test it.

At first, she tried leaving part of what she liked least (in her case, the vegetable). Eventually, she extended her rule to other foods and soon learned to maintain her weight quite easily by leaving a large portion of those foods that were least nutritious and/or most conducive to weight gain.

Breaking stimulus-response patterns through either replacement or confrontation are two of the methods I recommend in the area of weight loss. Another is best described as a "time-stretch."

This method involves a lengthening of the period of time during which you consume your food. Rapid and gluttonous ingestion of food can indeed slake one's hunger, but as we have seen, overeating is seldom a response to true hunger, but rather to a variety of other stimuli. Eating very quickly is not a good idea for anyone, since it makes digestion difficult, but it is particularly contraindicated for dieters.

"Gobbling" food was a habit that I myself had to break. I was an eager student (the word "voracious" comes to mind), often staying in my classes or laboratories until the last minute, then wolfing down some food before my next appointment. I eventually realized that this method of eating was depriving me of the normal oral and visual satisfactions of the food and, therefore, leading to a desire for more.

Time-stretch techniques reverse this process and assure dieters of all the satisfactions of normal food consumption. The following are methods I found most successful for myself and my patients:

1. In the beginning, monitor the pace of your eating by counting the average number of times you masticate—chew—your food per mouthful. Consciously increase that number. If it is ten, stretch it to twenty or even thirty.

2. Drink water before but not during a meal. It has been found that liquid before a meal creates a sensation of fullness. During a meal, however, it is not as effective, and tends to deprive a dieter of eating pleasure.

3. Completely swallow each bit of food before you put more on your fork or spoon. (This is a certain pace-slower.)

4. Count to thirty between bites.

5. Cut your food into small pieces and eat each piece one at a time.

6. When you are eating alone, use the "wrong" hand, i.e., if you are right-handed, use your left hand.

7. Also when you are alone (or in a Chinese restaurant), use chopsticks. For Westerners, these utensils usually slow the pace of their food consumption.

8. When you feel a craving for a snack, set a timer for ten minutes. If, after the bell rings, the craving is still with you, eat the snack then. Most of my patients report that they find their food cravings evaporate over that short period of time. (Again, this is an interesting check on internal [hunger] versus external stimuli.)

9. A mental game: When you are dining with companions, set yourself the competitive goal of being the *slowest* eater. Pick up your eating utensil after everyone has already begun to eat; put it down after everyone has finished.

Punishment and reward systems are also part of behavioral modification theory and, as many parents have discovered in disciplining their children, rewards, for the most part, are more effective than punishments.

As you progress on the Southampton Diet, you will discover that a sense of well-being, mental balance and good health rewards you far beyond any material gift. If, however, it pleases you to arrange to buy a new dress or handbag at the end of a successful week of dieting, feel free to do so. The Southampton Diet is a life-changing program. The changes it facilitates are all in the direction of new happiness, success and joy in living. If, along the way, you choose the pleasure of a material reward, this is all to the good.

These are the "reward" techniques I've found to be most effective.

1. Positive reinforcement. Each time you resist a diet-breaking temptation, give yourself a reward. The reward might be money, an article of clothing or some special event you'd like to attend (a hit show perhaps, or concert). In other words, the reward can be anything but food.

2. Practice "contractual dieting." A young patient of mine seemed to have hit a plateau on our diet plan. She'd lost forty pounds but had started to put a few pounds back on, and I suspected that she had been eating food that was not on the diet. I also remembered that she had once spoken about buying an alligator handbag. She had wanted one since she was a girl, she had said, but the bag she liked was now priced at $750—far too much for this thrifty lawyer.

Our solution was to make a pact. At each visit, she promised to tell me how and when she had strayed from the diet. If she *had* eaten something forbidden, she was obliged to pay me five dollars. If she hadn't, she would pay *herself* ten dollars.

I think you can guess how the story ends. My friend much preferred paying herself ten dollars to paying me five dollars. She quickly returned to the diet plan—and was soon on her way to buying that expensive alligator bag and losing the final ten pounds of her weight-loss goal.

You can make a similar pact with your spouse or with a friend.

PUTTING IT IN WRITING

Normally, I don't suggest that my diet patients do a great deal of paperwork. Dieting can be difficult enough without functioning as your own recording secretary. But some men and women require the discipline of writing things down. If you are such a person, it should help if you keep a food diary, especially if you have reached the maintenance level of the diet.

Keep your food diary as follows: Every day, write down exactly what you have eaten, what you were doing while you were eating (watching TV, talking on the phone, reading a newspaper), who was with you while you were eating, the time of day at which you ate (snacks included), how hungry you were when you ate and any emotions you may have felt at the time.

Collate your food diary into a weekly log and you will undoubtedly notice that certain patterns emerge. Seeing these patterns in writing will help you recognize the particular stimuli that lead to your own eating response.

THE MIRROR OF TRUTH

A moment generally appears in the life of every dieter when all else fails, when the impulse to eat seems overwhelming. I have experienced this moment more than once and have found one technique that always succeeds in such moments of crisis (as long as they occur—as they usually do—*after* work hours).

When you feel that overwhelming urge to overeat, take off all your clothes and stand in front of a mirror. If you are distressed by what you see, if the naked truth hurts, your desire to lose weight will dominate your desire to overeat. If you still feel a need to devour some confection, try to eat it while you are standing nude in front of that mirror. Watch yourself consume every crumb. I've stood in front of that looking glass myself and have never progressed past the first bite of that forbidden food.

As we have seen, the problem of overweight is complex

and cannot be expected to yield to *one* system of attack. All four points of the program must be taken into account. With these behavioral modification techniques, you now have the final point in the Southampton Diet program. They will not, however, accomplish your goal by themselves. In order to fully achieve your weight-loss goal you must have the proper diet, psychologically and nutritionally balanced. This is what the Southampton Diet provides. Yet, in my years of working with weight (my own and others'), I've learned five fundamentals:

1. The taller you are, the faster you lose.
2. The fatter you are, the faster you lose.
3. The younger you are, the faster you lose.
4. The more active you are, the faster you lose.
5. The better you diet, the faster you lose.

Rule number 5 is the most important of all: The better you diet, the faster you lose. With the Southampton Diet, you have the world's finest weight-reduction plan—whether you're tall or short, fat or not so fat, young or old, active or sedentary.

Your readiness to begin this program—to change your life into one that is Southampton thin and happy forever—will be tested in the next chapter.

8

THE SOUTHAMPTON DIET CONTRACT

IF YOU ARE READING THIS for the first time, please do not read any further at this moment.

The next chapter provides the Southampton Diet itself, and before you begin it, there are several things I would like you to do.

First of all, do you feel hungry? Or, more specifically, do you feel a desire to go on a food binge of any kind? If so, please do so right now.

If that sounds like a strange request, please consider the following:

The Southampton Diet itself involves a "turning" that is more than just a turning of the page. It is a turning around of your mind and your life. It means a commitment to caring for yourself instead of punishing yourself, and of becoming and staying thin forever.

Therefore, before you make this commitment—before you take this major life-changing step—I want you to be sure of what you are doing. I want you to be ready and fully convinced that the new, revitalized you who will emerge from this diet is who you really want to be.

If, somewhere in your mind, the suspicion lingers that food binges are truly valuable for you, that they are caring rather than self-punishing episodes, then please proceed to indulge in them right now. When you have had enough, please begin Chapter 1 of this book again. By the time you reach this point in the book the second time, you may be ready to read further.

These instructions are exactly the same as those I give my patients at the end of our initial interview. I ask them, as I am asking you, to think hard about all they have learned, even to return to the office again before they begin the diet if they have any further questions. Their understanding of the principles of the Southampton Diet is essential. And so is yours.

I recommend, in fact, that even if you have no desire to binge, you reread this book from the beginning anyway. Read it this time with your own personality traits and character in mind. As you complete each chapter, ask yourself if you have read anything in it that directly applies to you. Have you had difficulties with other diets? Perhaps you have experienced some of the problems you read about in Chapter 2. Have you developed a Fat Shield? Perhaps you recognize the emotional dynamic described in Chapter 3.

In one sense, you, as a reader, have an advantage over those of my patients who did not have this book. You can, in a leisurely fashion, examine every principle of the Southampton Diet at your own pace, on the printed page.

Please do so. Please be sure that you agree with most of these principles. Please note the ones that apply to you. Only when you have done this will you be ready to begin the Southampton Diet. And only when you're ready to begin the Southampton Diet will you also be prepared to enter a psychological contract with me.

What is that contract?

It is exactly the one I insist on with every one of my patients. You will find it below, and I hope that you, like each one of them, will consider it to be in your best interest to sign it, too. It is nothing more nor less than your commitment to becoming Southampton thin.

I understand that The Southampton Diet is a healthy, balanced, energizing plan specially designed by Stuart M. Berger, M.D., M.P.H. I hereby commit myself to it for a minimum of the next two weeks.

*(Signed)*_____

Now perhaps you would like a signed contract from me as well.

Here it is:

I guarantee that The Southampton Diet is specially balanced to provide a healthy, rapid weight loss to anyone who stays on it for two weeks or more. I also hope that you—as well as every other reader of this book—will refer to it often and draw from it the sense that I am with you in spirit every day of the program.

*(Signed)*_____
Stuart M. Berger, M.D., M.P.H.

THE
DIETS

The Southampton Diet Menu

WELCOME TO THE SOUTHAMPTON DIET PROGRAM

IF YOU GLANCE THROUGH THE NEXT FEW PAGES, you will see that the Southampton Diet is very simple to follow. No special preparations are needed and no extensive or obscure shopping is required. In addition to the diet plan as written, you may eat unlimited quantities of the following foods:

Chicory	Parsley
Celery cabbage (referred to as "Chinese cabbage" in most supermarkets)	Radishes
	Watercress
	Decaffeinated coffee
	Herb tea
Cucumbers	Mineral water
Endive	Seltzer
Escarole	Club soda
Lettuce (all varieties)	Lemon and lime juice

Suggestions for methods of cooking foods without using fats (such as for broiling or baking fish and chicken, poach-

109

ing chicken and turkey breasts for sandwiches and salads and boiling rice) are provided in the recipe section.

During Week 1 of the diet, you must follow the menus as written unless you are dining in a restaurant. In that case, you may substitute the appropriate meal from the Southampton Restaurant and Vacation Menu. After that meal, continue with the next snack or meal on Week 1. You may also substitute ½ cup of V-8 or tomato juice for the vegetables at any meal and ½ cup of unsweetened fruit juice for fruit. There is a choice between two breakfasts every day for variety.

When mixed green salad or mixed salad greens are called for in the diet just use any quantity desired of the vegetables listed on page 109.

It is important not to skip a meal or snack on the diet. The Southampton Diet is carefully balanced to provide not only proper nutrition but the correct distribution of amino acids and carbohydrates, as well as the glucose (sugar) and vitamins needed for the happy stress-free dieting as described in Chapters 4 and 5. The timing of when you consume your food is also important, so be sure to follow the menus as written, and eat snacks 2 to 3 hours after a meal.

If, for some reason, you forget to eat a snack, add it to the following meal. Do not, however, do this on a regular basis. And do not neglect your evening snack. Again, it is this special balance and timing of eating that will reduce anxiety and elevate mood, helping you to feel better as you lose weight.

You may even drink eight ounces of dry white wine weekly. I suggest that you occasionally mix an ounce or two with club soda (or any bottled water of your choice) to make a spritzer. Although mineral water is not included as a beverage on the breakfast menu, it is perfectly acceptable to drink it instead of decaffeinated coffee or herb tea.

Weigh your food portions (after cooking) on a postal scale for the first two or three days only. Also, measure starches and vegetables (after cooking) during this time. A set of graduated stainless steel or glass (Pyrex) measuring cups from ¼ cup to 2 cups would be most helpful. Vegetables can be cut into pieces to fit into the cups. After that, your eye will be trained and an estimate will be satisfactory.

When you have completed Week 1, begin Week 2. You can substitute any meal or snack from one or another of the ethnic diets for any meal or snack on the Week 2 menu. You will thus be able to enjoy a wide variety of delicious food while remaining within the carefully balanced parameters of the Southampton Diet.

Stay on this liberalized Week 2 plan until you have lost all the weight you care to lose. To *keep* your weight at this level—to be thin and happy for the rest of your life—follow the Southampton Maintenance Diet and reread Chapter 7 on behavioral techniques.

SHOPPING TIPS

Turkey, cottage cheese, skim milk and yogurt are eaten frequently on the Southampton Diet, in meals as well as snacks. Fruits such as pineapple or bananas are also consumed daily. I suggest that you purchase these foods in quantity. *All* fruits should be the smallest size available.

Fruits and vegetables have greater nutritive value and fiber content if they are fresh. I recommend that you purchase frozen vegetables and fruits or canned fruits (unsweetened, packed in their own juice, juice drained) only if fresh are unavailable.

All varieties of bran cereals are acceptable as long as no sugar has been added. Any kind of whole-grain bread or whole-wheat bread is fine.

All canned tuna fish should be packed in water (not oil) and drained before using. Canned salmon, crabmeat and shrimp are generally packed in brine, so simply drain them before using. I suggest that only white meat chicken be used in the diet, and that the skin be removed before cooking or eating. If you are roasting an entire turkey for a week's worth of meals, eat only the breast meat and not the drumsticks, thighs and other dark meat parts or the skin. Choose lean cuts of meat and remove all visible fat. Any kind of veal chop (such as loin, shoulder or rib) can be eaten—only breast of veal is off limits since it's quite fatty. Any kind of fish is fine.

Read the labels on cans or packages carefully to avoid unnecessary sugar or additives, including monosodium glutamate (MSG).

Avoid commercial salad dressings. Use the recipes for salad dressings that contain no oil, which are included in the recipe section, squeeze on lemon juice or add some vinegar and any herbs or spices of your choice.

Beverages containing caffeine (coffee, tea, some diet sodas) are not recommended because of their tendency to produce anxiety. However, drinking them will not inhibit your weight loss on the diet. If you haven't a preference for black coffee, you may add 2 tablespoons of skim milk to your decaffeinated coffee, if desired, but no sugar, cream or half and half. Although artificial sweeteners don't contain any substances that will affect your weight loss, they do have chemicals that some evidence suggests are unhealthy. I suggest that you avoid adding them to your food, if at all possible.

COOKING TIPS

With the exception of salt, which should be used only moderately in cooking and not added to a finished dish, food can be liberally seasoned. Any herbs or spices (not containing salt and sugar) can be used for flavoring. Basil, bay leaf, cayenne pepper, chili powder, cumin, curry powder, dill, fennel, garlic, ginger, horseradish, marjoram, mint, mustard (prepared or dried), onion powder, oregano, paprika, parsley, pepper, rosemary, sage, tarragon, and thyme are some that will add zest to your cooking. Avoid any condiments such as catsup, which are prepared with sugar.

Choose lean cuts of meat and remove all visible fat.

Suggestions for methods of cooking foods without additional fats are in "The Southampton Diet Recipes" chapter. Food can also be charcoal broiled for greater flavor. Use nonstick cooking utensils. Baste frequently and liberally with lemon or tomato juice (up to ½ cup a serving) or beef, chicken, vegetable, fish or veal stock to keep your low-fat meat juicy and moist. When sautéeing food (especially onions and mushrooms) add a few tablespoons of water or stock to prevent burning and sticking.

Whip 1 tablespoon of low-fat cottage cheese (perhaps with 1 teaspoon of low-fat buttermilk or yogurt added to make it smoother) and ½ to 1 teaspoon of chopped chives for a baked potato topping.

The herb tea and decaffeinated coffee can be brewed, chilled in the refrigerator and then poured over ice cubes. Garnish the tea with fresh mint and lemon wedges or slices and the coffee with a cinnamon stick for an attractive presentation.

You'll find that food prepared this way will have a clean, fresh taste. And you may enjoy it so much that it will inspire you to use these recipes even after you've lost your desired weight and have embarked on the Maintenance Diet. Through them you will learn to cook meals that are both exciting and healthful.

NOTE: Recipes for all menu items followed by an asterisk (*) can be found in "The Southampton Diet Recipes" section.

For your convenience, there follows a listing of the breakfasts (there is a choice of two) and the snacks included in Weeks 1 and 2 of the diet.

BREAKFASTS

BREAKFAST I	Unsweetened pineapple (½ cup)
	2% milk-fat cottage cheese (¼ cup)
	Whole-grain bread (1 slice)
	Decaffeinated coffee, herb tea

OR

BREAKFAST II	Banana (½)
	Skim milk (1 cup)
	Bran cereal (½ cup)
	Decaffeinated coffee, herb tea

SNACKS

	Afternoon Snack	Evening Snack
DAY 1	Turkey breast (1 ounce)	Plain low-fat yogurt (1 cup)
DAY 2	Plain low-fat yogurt (1 cup)	Banana (½)
DAY 3	Tomato juice (½ cup) and raw carrot sticks (½ cup)	Skim milk (1 cup)
DAY 4	2% milk-fat cottage cheese (¼ cup)	Plain low-fat yogurt (1 cup)
DAY 5	Apple (1)	Skim milk (1 cup)
DAY 6	2% milk-fat cottage cheese (¼ cup)	Plain low-fat yogurt (1 cup)
DAY 7	Orange (1)	Skim milk (1 cup)

Wine (8 ounces dry white wine per week)

SOUTHAMPTON DIET MENU

WEEK 1   DAY 1

BREAKFAST I   Unsweetened pineapple (½ cup)
2% milk-fat cottage cheese (¼ cup)
Whole-grain bread (1 slice)
Decaffeinated coffee, herb tea

OR

BREAKFAST II   Banana (½)
Skim milk (1 cup)
Bran cereal (½ cup)
Decaffeinated coffee, herb tea

LUNCH   *Open-face sandwich of*: sliced Cooked
Turkey breast* (2 ounces), sliced tomato
(½ cup), sliced cucumber (unlimited),
whole-wheat bread (1 slice)
Apple (1)
Decaffeinated coffee, herb tea, mineral
water

AFTERNOON SNACK   Turkey breast* (1 ounce)

DINNER   Broiled veal chop (4 ounces)
Brown Rice* (½ cup)
Steamed Zucchini* (½ cup)
Mixed green salad (unlimited)
Dressing* (unlimited)
Pear (1)
Decaffeinated coffee, herb tea, mineral
water

EVENING SNACK   Plain low-fat yogurt (1 cup)

115

SOUTHAMPTON DiET MENU

WEEK 1   DAY 2

BREAKFAST I   Unsweetened pineapple (½ cup)
2% milk-fat cottage cheese (¼ cup)
Whole-grain bread (1 slice)
Decaffeinated coffee, herb tea

OR

BREAKFAST II   Banana (½)
Skim milk (1 cup)
Bran cereal (½ cup)
Decaffeinated coffee, herb tea

LUNCH   *Southampton Salad Bowl of:* chopped hard-cooked egg (1), julienned Swiss cheese (1 ounce), tomato wedges (¼ cup), green pepper (¼ cup), sliced cucumber and mixed salad greens (unlimited)
Dressing* (unlimited)
Whole-wheat bread (1 slice)
Cantaloupe (¼)
Decaffeinated coffee, herb tea, mineral water

AFTERNOON   Plain low-fat yogurt (1 cup)
SNACK

DINNER   Broiled Chicken Breast* (4 ounces)
Baked potato (1 small)
Steamed Broccoli* (½ cup)
Mixed green salad
Dressing* (unlimited)
Strawberries (¾ cup)
Decaffeinated coffee, herb tea, mineral water

EVENING   Banana (½)
SNACK

116

SOUTHAMPTON DIET MENU

BREAKFAST I Unsweetened pineapple (½ cup)
2% milk-fat cottage cheese (¼ cup)
Whole-grain bread (1 slice)
Decaffeinated coffee, herb tea

OR

BREAKFAST II Banana (½)
Skim milk (1 cup)
Bran cereal (½ cup)
Decaffeinated coffee, herb tea

LUNCH *Southampton Salad Bowl of:* tuna (½ cup,
canned), sliced tomato (½ cup), raw onion
slice, sliced cucumber and mixed salad
greens (unlimited)
Dressing* (unlimited)
Rye bread (1 slice)
Honeydew melon (⅛)
Decaffeinated coffee, herb tea, mineral
water

AFTERNOON SNACK Tomato juice (½ cup)
Raw carrot sticks (½ cup)

DINNER Roast turkey breast* (4 ounces)
Brown Rice* (½ cup)
Steamed Summer Squash* (½ cup)
Mixed green salad (unlimited)
Dressing* (unlimited)
Orange (1)
Decaffeinated coffee, herb tea, mineral
water

EVENING SNACK Skim milk (1 cup)

117

SOUTHAMPTON DIET MENU

WEEK 1   DAY 4

BREAKFAST I   Unsweetened pineapple (½ cup)
2% milk-fat cottage cheese (¼ cup)
Whole-grain bread (1 slice)
Decaffeinated coffee, herb tea

OR

BREAKFAST II   Banana (½)
Skim milk (1 cup)
Bran cereal (½ cup)
Decaffeinated coffee, herb tea

LUNCH   *Open-face sandwich of*: Muenster cheese
(2 ounces), sliced tomato (½ cup), sliced
cucumber (unlimited), romaine lettuce
(unlimited), whole-wheat bread (1 slice)
Grapefruit (½)
Decaffeinated coffee, herb tea, mineral
water

AFTERNOON   2% milk-fat cottage cheese (¼ cup)
SNACK

DINNER   Baked Fish* (4 ounces)
Baked potato (1 small)
Steamed Carrots* (½ cup)
Mixed green salad (unlimited)
Dressing* (unlimited)
Peach (1)
Decaffeinated coffee, herb tea, mineral
water

EVENING   Plain low-fat yogurt (1 cup)
SNACK

SOUTHAMPTON DIET MENU

WEEK 1 DAY 5

BREAKFAST I
Unsweetened pineapple (½ cup)
2% milk-fat cottage cheese (¼ cup)
Whole-grain bread (1 slice)
Decaffeinated coffee, herb tea

OR

BREAKFAST II
Banana (½)
Skim milk (1 cup)
Bran cereal (½ cup)
Decaffeinated coffee, herb tea

LUNCH
Southampton Salad Bowl of: julienned
Cooked Turkey Breast* (1 ounce),
julienned Swiss cheese (1 ounce), tomato
wedges (½ cup), sliced cucumber and
mixed salad greens (unlimited)
Dressing* (unlimited)
Whole-wheat bread (1 slice)
Pear (1)
Decaffeinated coffee, herb tea, mineral
water

AFTERNOON SNACK
Apple (1)

DINNER
Lean roast beef (4 ounces)
Baked potato (1 small)
Steamed Brussels Sprouts* (½ cup)
Mixed green salad
Dressing* (unlimited)
Unsweetened pineapple (½ cup)
Decaffeinated coffee, herb tea, mineral
water

EVENING SNACK
Skim milk (1 cup)

119

SOUTHAMPTON DIET MENU

WEEK 1   DAY 6

BREAKFAST I Unsweetened pineapple (½ cup)
2% milk-fat cottage cheese (¼ cup)
Whole-grain bread (1 slice)
Decaffeinated coffee, herb tea

OR

BREAKFAST II Banana (½)
Skim milk (1 cup), Bran cereal (½ cup)
Decaffeinated coffee, herb tea

LUNCH *Southampton Salad Bowl of:* salmon (½ cup,
canned), sliced tomato (¼ cup), sliced
green pepper (¼ cup), sliced cucumber
and mixed salad greens (unlimited)
Dressing* (unlimited)
Whole-wheat bread (1 slice)
Pear (1)
Decaffeinated coffee, herb tea, mineral
water

AFTERNOON SNACK 2% milk-fat cottage cheese (¼ cup)

DINNER Broiled Fish* (4 ounces)
Brown Rice* (½ cup)
Steamed String Beans* (½ cup)
Mixed green salad (unlimited)
Dressing* (unlimited)
Unsweetened pineapple (½ cup)
Decaffeinated coffee, herb tea, mineral
water

EVENING SNACK Plain low-fat yogurt (1 cup)

SOUTHAMPTON DIET MENU

BREAKFAST I   Unsweetened pineapple (½ cup)
2% milk-fat cottage cheese (¼ cup)
Whole-grain bread (1 slice)
Decaffeinated coffee, herb tea

OR

BREAKFAST II   Banana (½)
Skim milk (1 cup)
Bran cereal (½ cup)
Decaffeinated coffee, herb tea

LUNCH   *Open-face sandwich of:* tuna (½ cup,
canned), sliced tomato (½ cup), sliced
cucumber (unlimited), Boston lettuce
(unlimited), rye bread (1 slice)
Cantaloupe (¼)
Decaffeinated coffee, herb tea, mineral
water

AFTERNOON SNACK   Orange (1)

DINNER   Baked Chicken Breast* (4 ounces)
Wild Rice* (½ cup)
Steamed Spinach* (½ cup)
Mixed green salad (unlimited)
Dressing* (unlimited)
Nectarine (1)
Decaffeinated coffee, herb tea, mineral
water

EVENING SNACK   Skim milk (1 cup)

121

SOUTHAMPTON DIET MENU

WEEK 2   DAY 1

BREAKFAST I   Unsweetened pineapple (½ cup)
2% milk-fat cottage cheese (¼ cup)
Whole-grain bread (1 slice)
Decaffeinated coffee, herb tea

OR

BREAKFAST II   Banana (½)
Skim milk (1 cup)
Bran cereal (½ cup)
Decaffeinated coffee, herb tea

LUNCH   *Stuffed pita sandwich of:* sliced Cooked
Turkey Breast* (2 ounces), sliced tomato
(½ cup), sliced cucumber and romaine
lettuce (unlimited), whole-wheat pita
bread (1 piece)
Apple (1)
Decaffeinated coffee, herb tea, mineral
water

AFTERNOON   Turkey breast* (1 ounce)
SNACK

DINNER   Broiled veal chop (4 ounces)
Brown Rice* (½ cup)
Steamed Zucchini* (½ cup)
Mixed green salad (unlimited)
Dressing* (unlimited)
Tangerine (1)
Decaffeinated coffee, herb tea, mineral
water

EVENING   Plain low-fat yogurt (1 cup)
SNACK

122

SOUTHAMPTON DIET MENU

WEEK 2   DAY 2

BREAKFAST I   Unsweetened pineapple (½ cup)
2% milk-fat cottage cheese (¼ cup)
Whole-grain bread (1 slice)
Decaffeinated coffee, herb tea

OR

BREAKFAST II   Banana (½)
Skim milk (1 cup)
Bran cereal (½ cup)
Decaffeinated coffee, herb tea

LUNCH   *Southampton Salad Bowl of:* 2% milk-fat
cottage cheese (½ cup), apple slices,
pineapple cubes, banana slices, grapefruit
sections (¼ cup of each), bed of lettuce
(unlimited)
Whole-wheat bread (1 slice)
Decaffeinated coffee, herb tea, mineral
water

AFTERNOON SNACK   Plain low-fat yogurt (1 cup)

DINNER   Broiled Chicken Breast* (4 ounces)
Baked winter squash (½ cup)
Sautéed mushrooms (½ cup)
Mixed green salad (unlimited)
Dressing* (unlimited)
Honeydew melon (⅛)
Decaffeinated coffee, herb tea, mineral
water

EVENING SNACK   Banana (½)

123

SOUTHAMPTON DIET MENU

WEEK 2   DAY 3

BREAKFAST I   Unsweetened pineapple (½ cup)
2% milk-fat cottage cheese (¼ cup)
Whole-grain bread (1 slice)
Decaffeinated coffee, herb tea

OR

BREAKFAST II   Banana (½)
Skim milk (1 cup)
Bran cereal (½ cup)
Decaffeinated coffee, herb tea

LUNCH   *Southampton Salad Bowl of:* baby shrimp
(2 ounces, or 10 shrimp), sliced tomato
(¼ cup), sliced green pepper (¼ cup),
mixed salad greens (unlimited)
Dressing* (unlimited)
Whole-wheat bread (1 slice)
Grapefruit (½)

**AFTERNOON
SNACK**   Tomato juice (½ cup)
Raw carrot sticks (½ cup)

DINNER   Roast turkey breast* (4 ounces)
Brown Rice* (½ cup)
Steamed Broccoli* (½ cup)
Mixed green salad (unlimited)
Dressing* (unlimited)
Cantaloupe (¼)
Decaffeinated coffee, herb tea, mineral
water

**EVENING
SNACK**   Skim milk (1 cup)

124

SOUTHAMPTON DIET MENU

WEEK 2   DAY 4

BREAKFAST I Unsweetened pineapple (½ cup)
2% milk-fat cottage cheese (¼ cup)
Whole-grain bread (1 slice)
Decaffeinated coffee, herb tea

OR

BREAKFAST II Banana (½)
Skim milk (1 cup)
Bran cereal (½ cup)
Decaffeinated coffee, herb tea

LUNCH *Open-face sandwich of:* sliced Cooked
Chicken Breast* (2 ounces), sliced tomato
(½ cup), sliced cucumber and romaine
lettuce (unlimited), whole-wheat bread (1
slice)
Pink grapefruit (½)

AFTERNOON SNACK 2% milk-fat cottage cheese (¼ cup)

DINNER Baked Fish* (4 ounces)
Brown Rice* (½ cup)
Steamed Asparagus Spears* (½ cup)
Mixed green salad (unlimited)
Dressing* (unlimited)
Unsweetened pineapple (½ cup)
Decaffeinated coffee, herb tea, mineral
water

EVENING SNACK Plain low-fat yogurt (1 cup)

125

SOUTHAMPTON DIET MENU

WEEK 2   DAY 5

BREAKFAST I   Unsweetened pineapple (½ cup)
2% milk-fat cottage cheese (¼ cup)
Whole-grain bread (1 slice)
Decaffeinated coffee, herb tea

OR

BREAKFAST II   Banana (½)
Skim milk (1 cup)
Bran cereal (½ cup)
Decaffeinated coffee, herb tea

LUNCH   *Southampton Salad Bowl of:* tuna (½ cup, canned), sliced tomato (¼ cup), sliced green pepper (¼ cup), sliced cucumber and mixed salad greens (unlimited)
Dressing* (unlimited)
Rye bread (1 slice)
Orange (1)
Decaffeinated coffee, herb tea, mineral water

AFTERNOON SNACK   Apple (1)

DINNER   Lean roast beef (4 ounces)
Baked potato (1 small)
Steamed Spinach* (½ cup)
Mixed green salad (unlimited)
Dressing* (unlimited)
Strawberries (¾ cup)
Decaffeinated coffee, herb tea, mineral water

EVENING SNACK   Skim milk (1 cup)

SOUTHAMPTON DIET MENU

BREAKFAST I   Unsweetened pineapple (½ cup)
2% milk-fat cottage cheese (¼ cup)
Whole-grain bread (1 slice)
Decaffeinated coffee, herb tea

OR

BREAKFAST II   Banana (½)
Skim milk (1 cup)
Bran cereal (½ cup)
Decaffeinated coffee, herb tea

LUNCH   *Southampton Salad Bowl of:* shredded
Cooked Chicken Breast* (2 ounces),
sliced tomato (¼ cup), sliced green pepper
(¼ cup), sliced cucumber and mixed salad
greens (unlimited)
Dressing* (unlimited)
Whole-wheat bread (1 slice)
Nectarine (1)
Decaffeinated coffee, herb tea, mineral
water

**AFTERNOON
SNACK**   2% milk-fat cottage cheese (¼ cup)

DINNER   Broiled Fish* (4 ounces)
Brown Rice* (½ cup)
Steamed Brussels Sprouts* (½ cup)
Mixed green salad (unlimited)
Dressing* (unlimited)
Grapefruit (½)
Decaffeinated coffee, herb tea, mineral
water

**EVENING
SNACK**   Plain low-fat yogurt (1 cup)

SOUTHAMPTON DIET MENU

BREAKFAST I   Unsweetened pineapple (½ cup)
2% milk-fat cottage cheese (¼ cup)
Whole-grain bread (1 slice)
Decaffeinated coffee, herb tea

OR

BREAKFAST II   Banana (½)
Skim milk (1 cup)
Bran cereal (½ cup)
Decaffeinated coffee, herb tea

LUNCH   *Open-face sandwich of:* sliced lean roast beef
(2 ounces), sliced tomato (½ cup), sliced
cucumber and lettuce (unlimited), whole-
wheat bread (1 slice)
Pear (1)
Decaffeinated coffee, herb tea, mineral
water

**AFTERNOON
SNACK**   Orange (1)

DINNER   Baked Chicken Breast* (4 ounces)
Wild Rice* (½ cup)
Steamed Cauliflower* (½ cup)
Mixed green salad (unlimited)
Dressing* (unlimited)
Cantaloupe (¼)

**EVENING
SNACK**   Skim milk (1 cup)

The Southampton Restaurant and Vacation Menu

EATING IN RESTAURANTS or hotel dining rooms while on vacation need pose no problems for the Southampton dieter.

When you are on vacation you can follow the menu plans you find here. Any meal can be interchanged with the appropriate prescribed meal from another day—the first day's for the third day's dinner meal, for instance.

The following guidelines will assure that you adhere to the Southampton Diet when you are dining outside your own home. They apply to occasional visits to restaurants as well as extended vacation trips (or even dinner parties).

1. Familiarize yourself with your diet plan before you leave home so that you will be aware of the proper amount and type of food to order.

2. Speak with the waiter or the chef about the method of cooking and the ingredients to be used. Ask him or her if food can be prepared according to your directions. Request that bread be brought to the table when the food is served, not before.

3. Avoid all cream soups, sauces or gravies.

4. Order only broiled, baked, steamed or poached food.

5. Remove all visible fat from meat and skin from poultry.

6. Ask that all butter, margarine or oils be eliminated in cooking or garnishing your meat. You can add pepper or other spices but avoid extra salt.

7. Remind your waiter not to put dressing on your salad. You may use lemon juice or vinegar or, if you like, bring your own jar of Southampton salad dressing.

8. Request fresh or unsweetened canned fruit for dessert.

9. Drink plain water, club soda or mineral water (with slice of lemon or lime).

10. If you are having an alcoholic drink before dinner, be sure your white wine or spritzer is within the week's eight-ounce limit.

SUBSTITUTIONS

When you are traveling or eating out, you will find, more often than not, that one or another of the Southampton restaurant meals is available. On those rare occasions when none of those meals can be obtained, this list of substitutes will be helpful.

• Two packages (4 slices) of melba toast = 1 slice whole-grain bread.

• ½ grapefruit = ½ banana = ¼ cantaloupe = ½ cup unsweetened fruit salad = ⅛ honeydew melon = ½ mango = 1 whole orange = 1 apple = ¾ cup strawberries = 1 peach = 1 pear.

• 4 ounces chicken = 4 ounces turkey = 4 ounces fish = 4 ounces veal = 5 medium shrimp or 10 small shrimp.

• Any vegetable can be substituted for another except these "sad" food vegetables: lima beans, peas, any dried beans.

• ½ cup unsweetened fruit juice = any prescribed fruit portion.

• ½ cup tomato or vegetable juice = any prescribed vegetable portion.

RESTAURANT AND VACATION MENU

BREAKFAST I   Unsweetened pineapple (½ cup) or
grapefruit (½)
2% milk-fat cottage cheese (¼ cup)
Whole-wheat toast (1 slice)
Decaffeinated coffee, herb tea

OR

BREAKFAST II   Banana (½) or cantaloupe (¼)
Skim milk (1 cup), Bran cereal (½ cup)
Decaffeinated coffee, herb tea

LUNCH   *Tuna plate of*: tuna (½ cup, canned), sliced
tomato (¼ cup), sliced green pepper
(¼ cup), sliced cucumber (unlimited), bed
of lettuce (unlimited)
Melba toast (4 slices)
Honeydew melon (⅛)
Decaffeinated coffee, herb tea, mineral
water

AFTERNOON SNACK   Turkey breast (1 ounce)

DINNER   Broiled chicken (4 ounces)
Rice (½ cup)
Steamed broccoli (½ cup)
Mixed green salad (unlimited), lemon wedge
or vinegar
Fresh fruit salad (½ cup)
Decaffeinated coffee, herb tea, mineral
water

EVENING SNACK   Plain low-fat yogurt (1 cup)

RESTAURANT AND VACATION MENU

DAY 2

BREAKFAST I Unsweetened pineapple (½ cup) or
grapefruit (½)
2% milk-fat cottage cheese (¼ cup)
Whole-wheat toast (1 slice)
Decaffeinated coffee, herb tea

OR

BREAKFAST II Banana (½) or cantaloupe (¼)
Skim milk (1 cup)
Bran cereal (½ cup)
Decaffeinated coffee, herb tea

LUNCH *Open-face sandwich of:* sliced turkey breast
(2 ounces), sliced tomato (½ cup), lettuce
(unlimited), whole-wheat bread (1 slice)
Unsweetened apple juice (½ cup)
Decaffeinated coffee, herb tea, mineral
water

AFTERNOON SNACK Plain low-fat yogurt (1 cup)

DINNER Baked fish (4 ounces)
Baked potato (1 small)
Zucchini (½ cup)
Mixed green salad (unlimited), lemon wedge
or vinegar
Grapefruit (½)
Decaffeinated coffee, herb tea, mineral
water

EVENING SNACK Banana (½)

RESTAURANT AND VACATION MENU

DAY 3

BREAKFAST I   Unsweetened pineapple (½ cup) or
grapefruit (½)
2% milk-fat cottage cheese (¼ cup)
Whole-wheat toast (1 slice)
Decaffeinated coffee, herb tea

OR

BREAKFAST II   Banana (½) or cantaloupe (¼)
Skim milk (1 cup)
Bran cereal (½ cup)
Decaffeinated coffee, herb tea

LUNCH   *Chef salad of:* julienned turkey breast (1
ounce), julienned Swiss cheese (1 ounce),
sliced tomato (¼ cup), sliced green pepper
(¼ cup), sliced cucumber (unlimited),
lettuce (unlimited)
Dressing* (unlimited)
Melba toast (4 slices)
Fresh fruit salad (½ cup)
Decaffeinated coffee, herb tea, mineral
water

AFTERNOON   Tomato juice (½ cup)
SNACK   Raw carrot sticks (½ cup)

DINNER   Broiled veal chop (4 ounces)
Rice (½ cup), String beans (½ cup)
Mixed green salad (unlimited), lemon wedge
or vinegar
Honeydew melon (⅛)
Decaffeinated coffee, herb tea, mineral
water

EVENING   Skim milk (1 cup)
SNACK

133

RESTAURANT AND VACATION MENU

DAY 4

BREAKFAST I   Unsweetened pineapple (½ cup) or
grapefruit (½)
2% milk-fat cottage cheese (¼ cup)
Whole-wheat toast (1 slice)
Decaffeinated coffee, herb tea

OR

BREAKFAST II   Banana (½) or cantaloupe (¼)
Skim milk (1 cup)
Bran cereal (½ cup)
Decaffeinated coffee, herb tea

LUNCH   *Fruit salad plate of:* 2% milk-fat cottage
cheese (¼ cup), unsweetened mixed fresh
fruit (any kind, 1 cup), bed of lettuce
(unlimited)
Melba toast (4 slices)
Decaffeinated coffee, herb tea, mineral
water

AFTERNOON SNACK   2% milk-fat cottage cheese (¼ cup)

DINNER   Broiled fish (4 ounces)
Rice (½ cup)
Asparagus spears (½ cup)
Mixed green salad (unlimited), lemon wedge
or vinegar
Fresh strawberries (¾ cup)
Decaffeinated coffee, herb tea, mineral
water

EVENING SNACK   Plain low-fat yogurt (1 cup)

RESTAURANT AND VACATION MENU

DAY 5

BREAKFAST I   Unsweetened pineapple (½ cup) or
grapefruit (½)
2% milk-fat cottage cheese (¼ cup)
Whole-wheat toast (1 slice)
Decaffeinated coffee, herb tea

OR

BREAKFAST II   Banana (½) or cantaloupe (¼)
Skim milk (1 cup), Bran cereal (½ cup)
Decaffeinated coffee, herb tea

LUNCH   Chilled shrimp cocktail (5 medium or 10
small shrimp) with horseradish and lemon
wedge
Bed of lettuce (unlimited)
Mixed raw carrots (¼ cup), celery (¼ cup)
and radishes (unlimited)
Melba toast (4 slices)
Grapefruit (½)
Decaffeinated coffee, herb tea, mineral
water

**AFTERNOON
SNACK**   Apple (1)

DINNER   Roast turkey breast (4 ounces)
Baked potato (1 small), Brussels sprouts (½ cup)
Mixed green salad (unlimited), lemon wedge
or vinegar
Cantaloupe (¼)
Decaffeinated coffee, herb tea, mineral
water

**EVENING
SNACK**   Skim milk (1 cup)

RESTAURANT AND VACATION MENU

DAY 6

BREAKFAST I   Unsweetened pineapple (½ cup) or
grapefruit (½)
2% milk-fat cottage cheese (¼ cup)
Whole-wheat toast (1 slice)
Decaffeinated coffee, herb tea

OR

BREAKFAST II   Banana (½) or cantaloupe (¼)
Skim milk (1 cup)
Bran cereal (½ cup)
Decaffeinated coffee, herb tea

LUNCH   *Open-face sandwich of*: sliced Swiss cheese
(2 ounces), sliced tomato (½ cup), lettuce
(unlimited), rye bread (1 slice)
Orange (1)
Decaffeinated coffee, herb tea, mineral
water

AFTERNOON SNACK   2% milk-fat cottage cheese (¼ cup)

DINNER   Clarified chicken consommé (1 cup)
Roast Cornish hen (4 ounces)
Rice (½ cup)
Broccoli (½ cup)
Mixed green salad (unlimited), lemon wedge
or vinegar
Fresh raspberries (½ cup) or fresh
strawberries (¾ cup)
Decaffeinated coffee, herb tea, mineral
water

EVENING SNACK   Plain low-fat yogurt (1 cup)

RESTAURANT AND VACATION MENU

DAY 7

BREAKFAST I   Unsweetened pineapple (½ cup) or
       grapefruit (½)
       2% milk-fat cottage cheese (¼ cup)
       Whole-wheat toast (1 slice)
       Decaffeinated coffee, herb tea

OR

BREAKFAST II   Banana (½) or cantaloupe (¼)
       Skim milk (1 cup), Bran cereal (½ cup)
       Decaffeinated coffee, herb tea

LUNCH   *Salmon plate of:* salmon (½ cup, canned),
       sliced tomato (¼ cup), sliced green pepper
       (¼ cup), slice of onion, sliced cucumber
       (unlimited), bed of lettuce (unlimited)
       Rye bread (1 slice)
       Grapefruit (½)
       Decaffeinated coffee, herb tea, mineral
       water

AFTERNOON SNACK   Orange (1)

DINNER   Steamed artichoke (1) with lemon juice
       Broiled lean steak (4 ounces filet mignon,
       tournedos, or London broil)
       Corn on the cob (1 ear)
       Mixed green salad (unlimited), lemon wedge
       or vinegar
       Blueberries, blackberries or raspberries (½ cup)
       Decaffeinated coffee, herb tea, mineral
       water

EVENING SNACK   Skim milk (1 cup)

THE
ETHNIC
DIETS

IF YOU HAVE COMPLETED the first week of the Southampton Diet you may begin either Week 2 or any of the ethnic menu plans that follow. You may also substitute a specific day's ethnic meal for the same day's meal on the Week 2 plan. The first day's lunch from the Italian or Jewish or French plan, for example, may replace the first day's lunch on the Week 2 plan.

These ethnic menus have been specially developed for people who enjoy and appreciate fine dining yet still want to lose weight. The variety is an important part of the pleasure you give yourself on the Southampton Diet.

You will find recipes for most of these authentic and delicious dishes in the recipes section of the book; dishes for which a recipe is given are marked with an asterisk (*).

I recommend these ethnic menus to you most highly and remind you again of the philosophy of the Southampton Diet program: Learn to stop punishing yourself and give yourself true pleasure instead.

For your convenience, there follows a listing of the breakfasts (there is a choice of two) and the snacks included in the ethnic diets.

141

BREAKFASTS

BREAKFAST I Unsweetened pineapple (½ cup)
2% milk-fat cottage cheese (¼ cup)
Whole-grain bread (1 slice)
Decaffeinated coffee, herb tea

OR

BREAKFAST II Banana (½)
Skim milk (1 cup)
Bran cereal (½ cup)
Decaffeinated coffee, herb tea

SNACKS

	Afternoon Snack	Evening Snack
Day 1	Turkey breast* (1 ounce)	Plain low-fat yogurt (1 cup)
Day 2	Plain low-fat yogurt (1 cup)	Banana (½)
Day 3	Tomato juice (½ cup) and raw carrot sticks (½ cup)	Skim milk (1 cup)
Day 4	2% milk-fat cottage cheese (¼ cup)	Plain low-fat yogurt (1 cup)
Day 5	Apple (1)	Skim milk (1 cup)
Day 6	2% milk-fat cottage cheese (¼ cup)	Plain low-fat yogurt (1 cup)
Day 7	Orange (1)	Skim milk (1 cup)

Wine (8 ounces dry white wine per week)

French and Nouvelle Cuisine Menu

ELEGANT NOUVELLE CUISINE is the most highly prized by the sophisticated residents of Southampton. This cuisine is the brilliant new development in French cooking that reflects the international concern for maintaining slim, healthy bodies. Eschewing the elaborate style and over-abundance of courses, sauces and rich ingredients in traditional French menus, it proposes instead new standards of excellence and freshness, clear, intense flavors and the preparation of beautiful plates in the kitchen rather than showy presentations at the table.

Not all nouvelle cuisine dishes are nonfattening, however, and the Southampton Diet program relies heavily on the work of one chef in particular—Michel Guerard—the inventor of the "cuisine minceur" of reduction and thinness. Guerard himself, at the age of forty-two, determined to "eat his way thin" and in doing so invented exciting new techniques and recipes. I am indebted to him for the basic thrust of many of the recipes included in this section as well as the principles which follow.

COOKING AND SHOPPING TIPS

• Buy and cook with foods that are the freshest in season and of excellent quality.

• Make presentation as important as cooking by creating geometric or other eye-pleasing patterns. Serve the new light sauces *under* rather than *poured over* the food.

• Experiment with new equipment on the market. Nonstick pans and food processors help eliminate the need for butter and oil in cooking.

• Free yourself from strict tradition. Be ready to try exotic ingredients and new combinations. Rediscover simple techniques such as poaching fish and pureeing vegetables.

• Learn to make intensely flavorful sauces by reducing, and thus thickening, stocks.

In the recipes that follow, advance preparation, careful measuring and the organization of tools remain as important as they ever were in traditional French cooking. But you will now have the opportunity to taste and enjoy sophisticated and delicious French food while continuing to lose weight on the Southampton Diet.

FRENCH AND NOUVELLE CUISINE MENU

DAY 1

BREAKFAST I   Unsweetened pineapple (½ cup)
2% milk-fat cottage cheese (¼ cup)
Whole-grain bread (1 slice)
Decaffeinated coffee, herb tea

OR

BREAKFAST II   Banana (½)
Skim milk (1 cup)
Bran cereal (½ cup)
Decaffeinated coffee, herb tea

LUNCH   Niçoise Salad* (½ cup tuna, ½ cup total of
vegetables)
Plain breadsticks (2)
Pear (1)
Decaffeinated coffee, herb tea, mineral
water

AFTERNOON SNACK   Turkey breast* (1 ounce)

DINNER   Poached Chicken Breasts Tarragon*
(4 ounces)
Cauliflower Puree* (½ cup)
Mixed green salad (unlimited)
Vinaigrette Dressing* (unlimited)
French bread (1 medium slice)
Strawberries and blueberries (½ cup total)
Decaffeinated coffee, herb tea, mineral
water

EVENING SNACK   Plain low-fat yogurt (1 cup)

FRENCH AND NOUVELLE CUISINE MENU

DAY 2

BREAKFAST I   Unsweetened pineapple (½ cup)
2% milk-fat cottage cheese (¼ cup)
Whole-grain bread (1 slice)
Decaffeinated coffee, herb tea

OR

BREAKFAST II   Banana (½)
Skim milk (1 cup)
Bran cereal (½ cup)
Decaffeinated coffee, herb tea

LUNCH   Cold Poached Chicken Breasts Tarragon*
(2 ounces)
Sautéed Snow Peas with Shallots and Basil*
(½ cup)
Plain breadsticks (2)
Unsweetened pineapple chunks (½ cup)
Decaffeinated coffee, herb tea, mineral
water

AFTERNOON SNACK   Plain low-fat yogurt (1 cup)

DINNER   Veal Pâté* (4 ounces)
Ratatouille* (½ cup)
Mixed green salad (unlimited)
Vinaigrette Dressing* (unlimited)
French bread (1 medium slice)
Sliced kiwi fruit and strawberries (½ cup)
Decaffeinated coffee, herb tea, mineral
water

EVENING SNACK   Banana (½)

FRENCH AND NOUVELLE CUISINE MENU

DAY 3

BREAKFAST I   Unsweetened pineapple (½ cup)
2% milk-fat cottage cheese (¼ cup)
Whole-grain bread (1 slice)
Decaffeinated coffee, herb tea

OR

BREAKFAST II   Banana (½)
Skim milk (1 cup)
Bran cereal (½ cup)
Decaffeinated coffee, herb tea

LUNCH   Cold Veal Pâté* (2 ounces)
Cold Ratatouille* (½ cup)
French bread (1 medium slice)
Strawberries (¾ cup)
Decaffeinated coffee, herb tea, mineral
water

AFTERNOON
SNACK   Tomato juice (½ cup)
Raw carrot sticks (½ cup)

DINNER   Baked Salmon Mousse* (⅔ cup)
Grilled Tomato with Rosemary*
(½ tomato)
Steamed Broccoli* (½ cup) (page 238)
Plain breadsticks (2)
Cantaloupe (¼) topped with 1 whole
strawberry
Decaffeinated coffee, herb tea, mineral
water

EVENING
SNACK   Skim milk (1 cup)

147

FRENCH AND NOUVELLE CUISINE MENU

DAY 4

BREAKFAST I   Unsweetened pineapple (½ cup)
2% milk-fat cottage cheese (¼ cup)
Whole-grain bread (1 slice)
Decaffeinated coffee, herb tea

OR

BREAKFAST II   Banana (½)
Skim milk (1 cup)
Bran cereal (½ cup)
Decaffeinated coffee, herb tea

LUNCH   Croque-Monsieur* (Melted Cheese
    Sandwich) (1 slice)
Cold Broccoli Vinaigrette* (½ cup)
Plums (2)
Decaffeinated coffee, herb tea, mineral
    water

AFTERNOON   2% milk-fat cottage cheese (¼ cup)
SNACK

DINNER   Steamed Fillet of Sole with Fennel*
    (4 ounces)
Rice (½ cup)
Steamed Asparagus* (½ cup) (page 238)
Poached Pears in Wine* (1)
Decaffeinated coffee, herb tea, mineral
    water

EVENING   Plain low-fat yogurt (1 cup)
SNACK

FRENCH AND NOUVELLE CUISINE MENU

DAY 5

BREAKFAST I
Unsweetened pineapple (½ cup)
2% milk-fat cottage cheese (¼ cup)
Whole-grain bread (1 slice)
Decaffeinated coffee, herb tea

OR

BREAKFAST II
Banana (½)
Skim milk (1 cup)
Bran cereal (½ cup)
Decaffeinated coffee, herb tea

LUNCH
Cold Steamed Fillet of Sole with Fennel*
  (2 ounces)
Cold Asparagus with Roquefort* (½ cup)
Plain breadsticks (2)
White grapes (12)
Decaffeinated coffee, herb tea, mineral
  water

AFTERNOON SNACK
Apple (1)

DINNER
Veau (Veal Cutlets) à la Provençale*
  (4 ounces)
Braised Leeks* (½ cup)
Mixed green salad (unlimited)
Vinaigrette Dressing* (unlimited)
French bread (1 medium slice)
Blueberries (½ cup)
Decaffeinated coffee, herb tea, mineral
  water

EVENING SNACK
Skim milk (1 cup)

FRENCH AND NOUVELLE CUISINE MENU

DAY 6

BREAKFAST I Unsweetened pineapple (½ cup)
2% milk-fat cottage cheese (¼ cup)
Whole-grain bread (1 slice)
Decaffeinated coffee, herb tea

OR

BREAKFAST II Banana (½)
Skim milk (1 cup), Bran cereal (½ cup)
Decaffeinated coffee, herb tea

LUNCH Onion Soup* (1 cup)
Sliced Tomatoes with Cucumber Sauce*
   (½ cup)
French bread (1 medium slice)
Sliced peach (1)
Decaffeinated coffee, herb tea, mineral
   water

**AFTERNOON
SNACK** 2% milk-fat cottage cheese (¼ cup)

DINNER Moules à la Marinière* (Mussels in Wine)
   (20 mussels)
Endive and watercress salad (unlimited) with
   sliced red pepper (½ cup)
Vinaigrette Dressing* (unlimited)
French bread (1 medium slice)
Blueberries and raspberries with fresh mint
   leaves (½ cup)
Decaffeinated coffee, herb tea, mineral
   water

**EVENING
SNACK** Plain low-fat yogurt (1 cup)

FRENCH AND NOUVELLE CUISINE MENU

DAY 7

BREAKFAST I   Unsweetened pineapple (½ cup)
2% milk-fat cottage cheese (¼ cup)
Whole-grain bread (1 slice)
Decaffeinated coffee, herb tea

OR

BREAKFAST II   Banana (½)
Skim milk (1 cup)
Bran cereal (½ cup)
Decaffeinated coffee, herb tea

LUNCH   Tomato juice (½ cup)
Fruit et Fromage* (Fruit and Cheese Plate)
   (1 pear, 2 ounces cheese)
French bread (1 medium slice)
Decaffeinated coffee, herb tea, mineral
   water

AFTERNOON   Orange (1)
SNACK

DINNER   Bouillabaisse* (Fish Stew) (4 ounces fish and
   seafood)
Gratin aux Zucchini* (Zucchini with
   Cheese) (½ cup)
Mixed green salad (unlimited)
Vinaigrette Dressing* (unlimited)
French bread (1 medium slice)
Poached Pears in Wine* (1)
Decaffeinated coffee, herb tea, mineral
   water

EVENING   Skim milk (1 cup)
SNACK

151

Italian Menu

MOST OF MY PATIENTS love Italian food, and a diet totally lacking in these robust Mediterranean flavors would be deprivation indeed.

The menus and recipes here have been specially developed to provide authentic Italian dining while you continue to lose weight on the Southampton Diet. You will find, to your surprise I'm sure, that pasta is included—though in smaller quantities than you may be used to eating. And there is even a recipe for pizza! Tomatoes, that essential ingredient, are used extensively in many of the recipes, especially for cooking meat and fish. Furthermore, the salad greens, which are such an integral part of Italian cuisine, may be eaten in unlimited quantities. Escarole, chicory, arugula, romaine and fennel, used so frequently in Italy, are good choices for the mixed green salads on the menus.

Coffee is included here as espresso (decaffeinated), and there is even a delicious recipe for cappuccino.

Since only small quantities of pasta are used, I suggest that you give yourself the pleasure of buying it fresh or a fine (dried), imported Italian brand such as De Cecco, made of pure Durham wheat. If you are allergic to wheat grains, you might try the Bolla products, which are produced from Jerusalem artichokes.

Both mineral water and wine are recommended throughout the Southampton Diet and since, in Italy, every well-set table features these beverages—either separately or mixed together—they are particularly appropriate here.

SHOPPING TIPS

• *Garlic:* Choose heads that are full and large, fresh and papery white. (Cook slowly to keep the flavor delicate and sweet.)
• *Cooking wine:* Buy good drinkable red or white wine. "Cooking" wines are too vinegary, and salt may have been added to them.

ITALIAN MENU

BREAKFAST I Unsweetened pineapple (½ cup)
2% milk-fat cottage cheese (¼ cup)
Whole-grain bread (1 slice)
Decaffeinated coffee, herb tea

OR

BREAKFAST II Banana (½)
Skim milk (1 cup)
Bran cereal (½ cup)
Decaffeinated coffee, herb tea

LUNCH Antipasto Salad* (1 ounce each of turkey
breast and skim-milk mozzarella, ½ cup
tomato wedges)
Plain breadsticks (2)
Honeydew melon (⅛)
Decaffeinated espresso, herb tea, mineral
water

AFTERNOON SNACK Turkey breast* (1 ounce)

DINNER Shrimp Marinara* (4 ounces)
Linguini (½ cup, cooked)
Steamed Italian Green Beans* (½ cup)
(page 238)
Plums (2)
Cappuccino,* decaffeinated espresso, herb
tea, mineral water

EVENING SNACK Plain low-fat yogurt (1 cup)

ITALIAN MENU

DAY 2

BREAKFAST I   Unsweetened pineapple (½ cup)
2% milk-fat cottage cheese (¼ cup)
Whole-grain bread (1 slice)
Decaffeinated coffee, herb tea

OR

BREAKFAST II Banana (½)
Skim milk (1 cup)
Bran cereal (½ cup)
Decaffeinated coffee, herb tea

LUNCH   Pizza Southampton* (1 slice)
Mixed green salad (unlimited)
Italian Dressing* (unlimited)
Peach (1)
Decaffeinated espresso, herb tea, mineral
    water

AFTERNOON SNACK   Plain low-fat yogurt (1 cup)

DINNER   Garlic Broiled Turkey* (4 ounces)
White Rice* (½ cup) (page 278)
Broccoli Salad* (½ cup)
Watermelon and cantaloupe balls (½ cup)
Cappuccino,* decaffeinated espresso, herb
    tea, mineral water

EVENING SNACK   Banana (½)

155

ITALIAN MENU

DAY 3

BREAKFAST I   Unsweetened pineapple (½ cup)
2% milk-fat cottage cheese (¼ cup)
Whole-grain bread (1 slice)
Decaffeinated coffee, herb tea

OR

BREAKFAST II   Banana (½)
Skim milk (1 cup)
Bran cereal (½ cup)
Decaffeinated coffee, herb tea

LUNCH   Tonno (Tuna) Salad* (2 ounces tuna, ½ cup
vegetables)
Breadsticks (2)
Pear (1)
Decaffeinated espresso, herb tea, mineral
water

AFTERNOON SNACK   Tomato juice (½ cup)
Raw carrot sticks (½ cup)

DINNER   Grilled Bluefish* (4 ounces)
Sliced Tomato Salad with Basil and
Oregano* (½ cup)
Whole-wheat Italian bread (1 medium slice)
Strawberries (¾ cup)
Cappuccino,* herb tea, mineral water

EVENING SNACK   Skim milk (1 cup)

156

ITALIAN MENU

BREAKFAST I   Unsweetened pineapple (½ cup)
2% milk-fat cottage cheese (¼ cup)
Whole-grain bread (1 slice)
Decaffeinated coffee, herb tea

OR

BREAKFAST II   Banana (½)
Skim milk (1 cup)
Bran cereal (½ cup)
Decaffeinated coffee, herb tea

LUNCH   Crostini* (Toasted Cheese Sandwich)
(1 slice)
Mixed green salad (unlimited)
Italian Dressing* (unlimited)
Honeydew melon (⅛)
Decaffeinated espresso, herb tea, mineral
water

AFTERNOON SNACK   2% milk-fat cottage cheese (¼ cup)

DINNER   Artichoke Salad* (1 artichoke)
Grilled Chicken* (4 ounces)
Linguini (½ cup, cooked) with Light Tomato
Sauce*
Blueberries (½ cup)
Cappuccino,* decaffeinated espresso, herb
tea, mineral water

EVENING SNACK   Plain low-fat yogurt (1 cup)

157

ITALIAN MENU

BREAKFAST I Unsweetened pineapple (½ cup)
2% milk-fat cottage cheese (¼ cup)
Whole-grain bread (1 slice)
Decaffeinated coffee, herb tea

OR

BREAKFAST II Banana (½)
Skim milk (1 cup)
Bran cereal (½ cup)
Decaffeinated coffee, herb tea

LUNCH Veal Burger* (2 ounces)
Mixed green salad (unlimited)
Italian Dressing* (unlimited)
Whole-wheat Italian bread (1 medium slice)
Nectarine (1)
Decaffeinated espresso, herb tea, mineral
water

AFTERNOON SNACK Apple (1)

DINNER Spigola Bollito (Poached Bass)* (4 ounces
fish, 2 new potatoes)
Roasted Red Pepper Salad* (½ cup)
Melon balls (½ cup)
Cappuccino,* decaffeinated espresso, herb
tea, mineral water

EVENING SNACK Skim milk (1 cup)

158

ITALIAN MENU

DAY 6

BREAKFAST I   Unsweetened pineapple (½ cup)
2% milk-fat cottage cheese (¼ cup)
Whole-grain bread (1 slice)
Decaffeinated coffee, herb tea

OR

BREAKFAST II   Banana (½)
Skim milk (1 cup)
Bran cereal (½ cup)
Decaffeinated coffee, herb tea

LUNCH   Cold Spigola Bollito (Cold Poached Bass)*
(2 ounces)
Arugula salad (¼ cup each sliced tomato
and Spanish onion, unlimited arugula)
Italian Dressing* (unlimited)
Plain breadsticks (2)
Pear (1)
Decaffeinated espresso, herb tea, mineral
water

AFTERNOON SNACK   2% milk-fat cottage cheese (¼ cup)

DINNER   Zuppa di Vongole or di Cozze (Clam or
Mussel Soup)* (20 small clams or mussels)
Green Bean Salad* (½ cup)
Whole-wheat Italian bread (1 medium slice)
Fruit Salad* (½ cup)
Cappuccino, * decaffeinated espresso, herb
tea, mineral water

EVENING SNACK   Plain low-fat yogurt (1 cup)

ITALIAN MENU

DAY 7

BREAKFAST I Unsweetened pineapple (½ cup)
2% milk-fat cottage cheese (¼ cup)
Whole-grain bread (1 slice)
Decaffeinated coffee, herb tea

OR

BREAKFAST II Banana (½)
Skim milk (1 cup), Bran cereal (½ cup)
Decaffeinated coffee, herb tea

LUNCH Sliced Tomatoes and Mozzarella Cheese
with Basil* (½ cup tomatoes, 2 ounces
cheese)
Arugula and chicory salad (unlimited)
Italian Dressing* (unlimited)
Whole-wheat Italian bread (1 medium slice)
Fresh fig (1)
Decaffeinated espresso, herb tea, mineral
water

AFTERNOON SNACK Orange (1)

DINNER Codfish Steaks in Tomato Sauce*
(4 ounces)
Linguini (½ cup, cooked)
Garlic-Flavored Spinach* (½ cup)
Blueberries (¼ cup) and strawberries
(½ cup)
Cappuccino,* decaffeinated espresso, herb
tea, mineral water

EVENING SNACK Skim milk (1 cup)

160

Japanese Menu

JAPANESE CUISINE IS particularly suited to the Southampton Diet because it is low in fat and consistently nutritionally sound.

Typically, Japanese cooking is efficient and well planned. Actual cooking time is short and much depends on careful preparation and artistic presentation. Each dish should be pleasing to the eye as well as the palate and should, according to Japanese tradition, contain at least two textures and three colors (red, green and either white or brown).

When you shop for the menus that follow, choose only the best ingredients—high-quality chicken, crisp, fresh young vegetables, good soy sauce (made without sugar and preferably the low-salt variety), the freshest fish, et cetera. (If you use frozen fish, defrost it slowly in milk to eliminate any fishy taste or smell.)

The following menus vary slightly from those you might find in a Japanese restaurant to conform to the diet, but none of the essential flavors have been lost in the process.

Preparation is not difficult, and many of the recipes will make a delicious change at mealtime.

COOKING AND SHOPPING TIPS

• *Dashi*: A delicate all-purpose stock and seasoning (traditionally made from dried fish flakes) used in Japan is replaced by chicken bouillon in these recipes. Whenever you are cooking chicken, just save pan juices; cool and then pour into a jar to chill in the refrigerator. The cooled hard fat can be separated from the jelled juices, then clarified. The jelly, with the addition of a little water, becomes dashi or chicken bouillon. A good variety of canned chicken broth (such as College Inn) will also work satisfactorily.

• *Disposable bamboo skewers:* Can be replaced with metal barbecue stakes, but cooking time will be much shorter, since the metal conducts heat.

• *Garnishes:* Alternatives are often given—parsley can be substituted when watercress is not in season; radishes, tomatoes or carrots are used for color.

• *Ginger juice:* Can be obtained by placing a small piece of ginger in a garlic press, which is then squeezed so that the juice can be extracted.

• *Light soy sauce:* Where recipes specifically call for light soy sauce, dark soy sauce may be substituted by mixing three-quarter parts dark sauce with one-quarter water.

• *Rice crackers and cakes (plain):* These are both produced commercially; the cakes are made of puffed rice and are packaged in cellophane wrappers. They can be found in Oriental grocery stores (and vegetable markets), food specialty shops and in most supermarkets.

• *Rice vinegar:* Inexpensive white cooking wine can be substituted.

• *Soy sauce:* Kikkoman is an excellent brand of soy sauce. The company produces light, dark and even low-salt varieties.

• *Sake:* A Japanese wine made from rice.

• *Toasted sesame seeds:* The sesame seeds one would purchase in a store are white in color, and plain. Toasting the seeds gives them a nutty flavor and crunchy texture. Since many of the recipes contain them (in small quantities), two methods for toasting sesame seeds are provided here:

1. Cook seeds in a saucepan over medium heat. Shake pan and stir continuously until golden colored, about 10 minutes. Remove from pan immediately. Cool.

2. Sprinkle the sesame seeds on a cookie sheet. Toast the

seeds for 10–15 minutes in a 350° F. oven or for 5 minutes under a hot broiler. Remove from sheet immediately. Cool.

Sesame seeds can be toasted in quantity, stored in a tightly covered jar and used as required.

JAPANESE MENU

DAY 1

BREAKFAST I   Unsweetened pineapple (½ cup)
2% milk-fat cottage cheese (¼ cup)
Whole-grain bread (1 slice)
Decaffeinated coffee, herb tea

OR

BREAKFAST II   Banana (½)
Skim milk (1 cup)
Bran cereal (½ cup)
Decaffeinated coffee, herb tea

LUNCH   Three-Flavor Vinegar Crab Salad* (½ cup crab)
Bed of lettuce or celery cabbage (unlimited)
Rice crackers (2)
Unsweetened Mandarin orange sections (½ cup)
Herb tea, mineral water

AFTERNOON SNACK   Turkey breast* (1 ounce)

DINNER   Chicken Teriyaki* (4 ounces chicken, ½ cup vegetables)
White Rice* (½ cup)
Simmered String Beans* (½ cup)
Watermelon and cantaloupe balls (½ cup)
Herb tea, mineral water

EVENING SNACK   Plain low-fat yogurt (1 cup)

164

JAPANESE MENU

DAY 2

BREAKFAST I   Unsweetened pineapple (½ cup)
2% milk-fat cottage cheese (¼ cup)
Whole-grain bread (1 slice)
Decaffeinated coffee, herb tea

OR

BREAKFAST II   Banana (½)
Skim milk (1 cup)
Bran cereal (½ cup)
Decaffeinated coffee, herb tea

LUNCH   Chicken and Asparagus Salad with Mustard
Dressing* (2 ounces chicken, ½ cup
vegetables)
Rice crackers (2)
Fresh apricots (2)
Herb tea, mineral water

AFTERNOON SNACK   Plain low-fat yogurt (1 cup)

DINNER   Sake Simmered Fish* (4 ounces)
White Rice* (½ cup)
Green Beans with Sesame Dressing*
(½ cup)
Fresh Bing cherries (10)
Herb tea, mineral water

EVENING SNACK   Banana (½)

165

JAPANESE MENU

DAY 3

BREAKFAST I   Unsweetened pineapple (½ cup)
2% milk-fat cottage cheese (¼ cup)
Whole-grain bread (1 slice)
Decaffeinated coffee, herb tea

OR

BREAKFAST II   Banana (½)
Skim milk (1 cup)
Bran cereal (½ cup)
Decaffeinated coffee, herb tea

LUNCH   Three-Flavor Vinegar Shrimp Salad*
(2 ounces shrimp)
Bed of lettuce or celery cabbage (unlimited)
Rice crackers (2)
Pink grapefruit (½)
Herb tea, mineral water

AFTERNOON SNACK   Tomato juice (½ cup)
Raw carrot sticks (½ cup)

DINNER   Chicken Yakitori with Vegetables*
(4 ounces chicken, ½ cup vegetables)
White Rice* (½ cup), topped with sliced
scallions
Sliced cucumbers (unlimited)
Sesame Dressing* (unlimited) (page 282)
Persimmon (1)
Herb tea, mineral water

EVENING SNACK   Skim milk (1 cup)

166

JAPANESE MENU

DAY 4

BREAKFAST I   Unsweetened pineapple (½ cup)
2% milk-fat cottage cheese (¼ cup)
Whole-grain bread (1 slice)
Decaffeinated coffee, herb tea

OR

BREAKFAST II   Banana (½)
Skim milk (1 cup)
Bran cereal (½ cup)
Decaffeinated coffee, herb tea

LUNCH   Chicken and Beansprout Salad with Sesame
Dressing* (2 ounces chicken, ½ cup
vegetables)
Bed of lettuce or celery cabbage (unlimited)
Rice crackers (2)
Pear (1)
Herb tea, mineral water

AFTERNOON SNACK   2% milk-fat cottage cheese (¼ cup)

DINNER   Scallops Yakitori with Vegetables*
(4 ounces scallops, ½ cup vegetables)
White Rice* (½ cup)
Sliced kiwi fruit (1)
Herb tea, mineral water

EVENING SNACK   Plain low-fat yogurt (1 cup)

JAPANESE MENU

DAY 5

BREAKFAST I Unsweetened pineapple (½ cup)
2% milk-fat cottage cheese (¼ cup)
Whole-grain bread (1 slice)
Decaffeinated coffee, herb tea

OR

BREAKFAST II Banana (½)
Skim milk (1 cup)
Bran cereal (½ cup)
Decaffeinated coffee, herb tea

LUNCH Tofu Salad* (2 ounces tofu, ½ cup
vegetables)
Sesame Dressing* (unlimited)
Rice crackers (2)
Tangerine (1)
Herb tea, mineral water

AFTERNOON SNACK Apple (1)

DINNER Mixed Grill Yakitori* (4 ounces total
chicken and shrimp, ½ cup vegetables)
White Rice* (½ cup)
Spinach with Sesame Dressing* (½ cup)
Unsweetened pineapple cubes (½ cup)
Herb tea, mineral water

EVENING SNACK Skim milk (1 cup)

JAPANESE MENU

DAY 6

BREAKFAST I   Unsweetened pineapple (½ cup)
2% milk-fat cottage cheese (¼ cup)
Whole-grain bread (1 slice)
Decaffeinated coffee, herb tea

OR

BREAKFAST II   Banana (½)
Skim milk (1 cup)
Bran cereal (½ cup)
Decaffeinated coffee, herb tea

LUNCH   Noodles with Broth* (1 cup broth, 2 ounces
     chicken, ½ cup cooked noodles)
Salad of: Bibb lettuce or celery cabbage
     (unlimited), thinly sliced tomato (½ cup)
     and thinly sliced cucumber (unlimited)
Sesame Dressing* (unlimited)
Orange (1)
Herb tea, mineral water

AFTERNOON SNACK   2% milk-fat cottage cheese (¼ cup)

DINNER   Fish Teriyaki* (4 ounces fish, ½ cup
     vegetables)
White Rice* (½ cup)
Sliced Radishes and Cucumbers with
     Sesame Dressing* (unlimited)
Persimmon (1)
Herb tea, mineral water

EVENING SNACK   Plain low-fat yogurt (1 cup)

JAPANESE MENU

DAY 7

BREAKFAST I Unsweetened pineapple (½ cup)
2% milk-fat cottage cheese (¼ cup)
Whole-grain bread (1 slice)
Decaffeinated coffee, herb tea

OR

BREAKFAST II Banana (½)
Skim milk (1 cup)
Bran cereal (½ cup)
Decaffeinated coffee, herb tea

LUNCH Chicken and Cucumber Salad with Sesame
Dressing* (2 ounces chicken)
Cucumbers (unlimited)
Bed of Boston lettuce (unlimited)
Rice crackers (2)
Herb tea, mineral water

AFTERNOON SNACK Orange (1)

DINNER Baked Fish with Mushrooms in a Package*
(4 ounces fish)
White Rice* (½ cup)
Simmered Carrots* (½ cup)
Honeydew melon (⅛)
Herb tea, mineral water

EVENING SNACK Skim milk (1 cup)

170

Chinese Menu

IT IS NOT SURPRISING that Chinese cooking has become so immensely popular in the United States. It is not only nutritious and light, but it also combines taste, texture and aroma in dishes that please the palate and refresh the senses.

The extensive use of vegetables, fish and lean meats in Chinese cuisine makes it happily amenable to the principles of the Southampton Diet. As a result, you will find quite a few of the traditional recipes here as well as several others you may not have tried in Chinese restaurants.

When you serve these delicious meals, or any of those you will find in the Japanese section, try using chopsticks and hot, scented towels to add to your dining pleasure.

SHOPPING TIPS

• *Snow peas:* They are now widely available in supermarkets. Look for fresh, green pods that are firm and contain very small peas. Trim ends and pull out the "string" before cooking.
• *Beansprouts:* Look for white, plump sprouts and avoid thin, brownish ones. Cover with water, keep in the refrigerator and change the water daily. They can keep for up to a week.
• *Bokchoy* (or Chinese cabbage). The long white stalks and green leaves are completely edible and the younger variety has yellow flowers which can also be eaten. This variety of cabbage (Chinese cabbage to the Chinese) can be bought primarily in Chinese markets in cities that have a Chinatown.

171

• *Celery cabbage:* This can be purchased in most supermarkets and is often sold as "Chinese cabbage" in American markets. It is used here in soups and salads with other ingredients. It is available in two varieties: the thick, short, round white head with light-green tops and the longer-stemmed, light-green cabbage with broad green leaves. Unless specified in a recipe, they are interchangeable.

• *Transparent noodles (also known as "cellophane noodles" or "vermicelli" bean threads):* These are made from green soybeans, starch and water. They are purchased in brittle bundles of opaque threads and should be soaked in hot water before you use them in soup.

• *Fermented black beans:* These are used to add that uniquely Chinese flavor to many meat and fish dishes such as the delicious steamed bass recipe you will find here. Black beans can be found in some supermarkets or in any local store that supplies Chinese restaurants. If they are not available in your area, the dish can be made without them.

• *Ginger:* The root is now available in many supermarkets and ethnic stores. Look for a hard, smooth-skinned surface, which indicates freshness and juiciness. It will keep for up to two weeks in the vegetable bin of your refrigerator. Fresh ginger can also be preserved for longer periods of time by cutting it in pieces and placing it in a screw-top jar, then covering it with dry sherry. Do not substitute powdered or dried ginger for fresh—it will not be as fragrant.

• *Rice cakes (plain):* These are made of puffed rice shaped into cakes. They can be purchased in Oriental grocery stores and vegetable markets, food specialty shops and in most supermarkets.

• *Soy sauce:* Use only the brands that do not contain added sugar, and preferably the new low-salt variety. Products recommended in the Japanese Menu section are best.

COOKING TIPS

Be sure that all ingredients are weighed, portioned and prepared in advance. Cooking time should usually be a matter of minutes and, in some cases, thirty seconds can make all the difference between succulent and burnt.

A nonstick electric or regular top-of-the-stove wok is the most efficient utensil to use for cooking these dishes. The deep sides of the wok help to cook the food faster and, therefore, keep it crisp. A nonstick skillet can be used, but it may not be as effective.

173

CHINESE MENU

BREAKFAST I Unsweetened pineapple (½ cup)
2% milk-fat cottage cheese (¼ cup)
Whole-grain bread (1 slice)
Decaffeinated coffee, herb tea

OR

BREAKFAST II Banana (½)
Skim milk (1 cup)
Bran cereal (½ cup)
Decaffeinated coffee, herb tea

LUNCH Peking Salad* (2 ounces chicken, ½ cup
vegetables)
Rice cakes (2)
Unsweetened Mandarin orange sections
(½ cup)
Herb tea, mineral water

**AFTERNOON
SNACK** Turkey breast* (1 ounce)

DINNER Steamed Sea Bass* (4 ounces)
White Rice* (½ cup) (page 278)
Stir-Fry Broccoli* (½ cup)
Unsweetened pineapple cubes (½ cup)
Herb tea, mineral water

**EVENING
SNACK** Plain low-fat yogurt (1 cup)

CHINESE MENU

BREAKFAST I   Unsweetened pineapple (½ cup)
2% milk-fat cottage cheese (¼ cup)
Whole-grain bread (1 slice)
Decaffeinated coffee, herb tea

OR

BREAKFAST II   Banana (½)
Skim milk (1 cup)
Bran cereal (½ cup)
Decaffeinated coffee, herb tea

LUNCH   Vermicelli Soup* (2 ounces chicken, ½ cup
noodles, 1 cup broth)
Chinese Vegetable Salad* (½ cup)
Nectarine (1)
Herb tea, mineral water

AFTERNOON SNACK   Plain low-fat yogurt (1 cup)

DINNER   Steamed Chicken* (4 ounces)
White Rice* (½ cup) (page 278)
Stir-Fry Carrots* (½ cup)
Spicy Cucumber Salad* (unlimited)
Persimmon (1)
Herb tea, mineral water

EVENING SNACK   Banana (½)

175

CHINESE MENU

BREAKFAST I Unsweetened pineapple (½ cup)
2% milk-fat cottage cheese (¼ cup)
Whole-grain bread (1 slice)
Decaffeinated coffee, herb tea

OR

BREAKFAST II Banana (½)
Skim milk (1 cup)
Bran cereal (½ cup)
Decaffeinated coffee, herb tea

LUNCH Peking Salad* (2 ounces shrimp, ½ cup
vegetables)
Rice cakes (2)
Apricots (2)
Herb tea, mineral water

AFTERNOON SNACK Tomato juice (½ cup)
Raw carrot sticks (½ cup)

DINNER Stir-Fry Chicken with Asparagus* (4 ounces
chicken, ½ cup vegetables)
White Rice* (½ cup) (page 278)
Pomegranate ("Chinese apple") (1)
Herb tea, mineral water

EVENING SNACK Skim milk (1 cup)

CHINESE MENU

DAY 4

BREAKFAST I   Unsweetened pineapple (½ cup)
2% milk-fat cottage cheese (¼ cup)
Whole-grain bread (1 slice)
Decaffeinated coffee, herb tea

OR

BREAKFAST II   Banana (½)
Skim milk (1 cup)
Bran cereal (½ cup)
Decaffeinated coffee, herb tea

LUNCH   Peking Salad* (2 ounces bean curd, ½ cup
vegetables)
Rice cakes (2)
Honeydew melon (⅛)
Herb tea, mineral water

AFTERNOON SNACK   2% milk-fat cottage cheese (¼ cup)

DINNER   Stir-Fry Shrimp with Snow Peas* (4 ounces
shrimp, ½ cup vegetables)
White Rice* (½ cup) (page 278)
Chinese Vegetable Salad* (½ cup)
Cherries (10)
Herb tea, mineral water

EVENING SNACK   Plain low-fat yogurt (1 cup)

CHINESE MENU

DAY 5

BREAKFAST I Unsweetened pineapple (½ cup)
2% milk-fat cottage cheese (¼ cup)
Whole-grain bread (1 slice)
Decaffeinated coffee, herb tea

OR

BREAKFAST II Banana (½)
Skim milk (1 cup)
Bran cereal (½ cup)
Decaffeinated coffee, herb tea

LUNCH Peking Salad* (½ cup salmon, ½ cup
vegetables)
Rice cakes (2)
Plums (2)
Herb tea, mineral water

**AFTERNOON
SNACK** Apple (1)

DINNER Steamed Red Snapper* (4 ounces)
Stir-Fry String Beans* (½ cup)
White Rice* (½ cup) (page 278)
Mango (½ cup)
Herb tea, mineral water

**EVENING
SNACK** Skim milk (1 cup)

CHINESE MENU

BREAKFAST I Unsweetened pineapple (½ cup)
2% milk-fat cottage cheese (¼ cup)
Whole-grain bread (1 slice)
Decaffeinated coffee, herb tea

OR

BREAKFAST II Banana (½)
Skim milk (1 cup)
Bran cereal (½ cup)
Decaffeinated coffee, herb tea

LUNCH Peking Salad* (½ cup crabmeat, ½ cup
vegetables)
Rice cakes (2)
Tangerine (1)
Herb tea, mineral water

AFTERNOON 2% milk-fat cottage cheese (¼ cup)
SNACK

DINNER Stir-Fry Scallops with Mushrooms and Red
Pepper* (4 ounces scallops, ½ cup
vegetables)
White Rice* (½ cup) (page 278)
Fresh or unsweetened canned kumquats (3)
Herb tea, mineral water

EVENING Plain low-fat yogurt (1 cup)
SNACK

CHINESE MENU

DAY 7

BREAKFAST I   Unsweetened pineapple (½ cup)
2% milk-fat cottage cheese (¼ cup)
Whole-grain bread (1 slice)
Decaffeinated coffee, herb tea

OR

BREAKFAST II   Banana (½)
Skim milk (1 cup)
Bran cereal (½ cup)
Decaffeinated coffee, herb tea

LUNCH   Peking Salad* (½ cup tuna, ½ cup
vegetables)
Rice cakes (2)
Peach (1)
Herb tea, mineral water

AFTERNOON SNACK   Orange (1)

DINNER   Stir-Fry Chicken (or Beef) with Broccoli*
(4 ounces chicken or beef, ½ cup vegetable)
White Rice* (½ cup) (page 278)
Spicy Cucumber Salad* (unlimited)
Pear (1)
Herb tea, mineral water

EVENING SNACK   Skim milk (1 cup)

180

Greek Menu

GREEK CUISINE—reflecting, as it does, the warmth and flavor of that hospitable country—is a welcome bit of sunshine in anyone's diet. Many of the recurring elements—lemons, yogurt, cucumbers, pita bread, and feta cheese; spices such as mint, basil, dill and oregano —add savory and pungent variety to meals.

The adaptations of Greek recipes which you find here have been specially designed in accordance with the Southampton Diet program. Seek and you shall find your favorite: Greek Salad, Dolmitas (stuffed grape leaves), and Mediterranean Fish Stew. The Chilled Cucumber-Yogurt Soup is a great favorite of Southamptonites returning from a hot day on the beach.

The ingredients used in the recipes are readily available, and the few that are not on supermarket shelves can be found in the delicatessens that supply local Greek, Turkish and Armenian communities in your area.

Commercial yogurt may not duplicate the firm, creamy consistency of homemade, but I have found the flavor almost exactly the same. Pour out the watery whey before measuring the quantities called for in these recipes.

181

GREEK MENU

DAY 1

BREAKFAST I   Unsweetened pineapple (½ cup)
2% milk-fat cottage cheese (¼ cup)
Whole-grain bread (1 slice)
Decaffeinated coffee, herb tea

OR

BREAKFAST II   Banana (½)
Skim milk (1 cup)
Bran cereal (½ cup)
Decaffeinated coffee, herb tea

LUNCH   Greek Salad I* (2 ounces feta, ½ cup total
vegetables)
Whole-wheat pita bread (1 piece)
Honeydew melon (⅛)
Decaffeinated coffee, herb tea, mineral
water

AFTERNOON SNACK   Turkey breast* (1 ounce)

DINNER   Shrimp Mykonos* (4 ounces)
Saffron Rice* (½ cup)
Eggplant Salad* (½ cup)
Green or black grapes (12)
Decaffeinated coffee, herb tea, mineral
water

EVENING SNACK   Plain low-fat yogurt (1 cup)

GREEK MENU

BREAKFAST I   Unsweetened pineapple (½ cup)
2% milk-fat cottage cheese (¼ cup)
Whole-grain bread (1 slice)
Decaffeinated coffee, herb tea

OR

BREAKFAST II   Banana (½)
Skim milk (1 cup)
Bran cereal (½ cup)
Decaffeinated coffee, herb tea

LUNCH   Grilled Feta Sandwich* (1)
Greek Salad II* (½ cup total vegetables)
Pear (1)
Decaffeinated coffee, herb tea, mineral
water

AFTERNOON   Plain low-fat yogurt (1 cup)
SNACK

DINNER   Baked Chicken with Lemon and Herbs*
(4 ounces)
Saffron Rice* (½ cup)
Steamed Spinach with Dill and Lemon*
(½ cup)
Dates (2)
Decaffeinated coffee, herb tea, mineral
water

EVENING   Banana (½)
SNACK

GREEK MENU

DAY 3

BREAKFAST I Unsweetened pineapple (½ cup)
2% milk-fat cottage cheese (¼ cup)
Whole-grain bread (1 slice)
Decaffeinated coffee, herb tea

OR

BREAKFAST II Banana (½)
Skim milk (1 cup)
Bran cereal (½ cup)
Decaffeinated coffee, herb tea

LUNCH Chicken Salad* (2 ounces chicken, ½ cup
vegetables)
Whole-wheat pita bread (1 piece)
Pear (1)
Decaffeinated coffee, herb tea, mineral
water

**AFTERNOON
SNACK** Tomato juice (½ cup)
Raw carrot sticks (½ cup)

DINNER Mediterranean Fish Stew* (4 ounces)
Saffron Rice* (½ cup)
Cucumber and Yogurt Salad* (½ cup)
Casaba melon (⅛)
Decaffeinated coffee, herb tea, mineral
water

**EVENING
SNACK** Skim milk (1 cup)

GREEK MENU

BREAKFAST I   Unsweetened pineapple (½ cup)
2% milk-fat cottage cheese (¼ cup)
Whole-grain bread (1 slice)
Decaffeinated coffee, herb tea

OR

BREAKFAST II   Banana (½)
Skim milk (1 cup)
Bran cereal (½ cup)
Decaffeinated coffee, herb tea

LUNCH   Tuna Salad* (½ cup tuna, ½ cup vegetables)
Whole-wheat pita bread (1 piece)
Apple (1)
Decaffeinated coffee, herb tea, mineral
water

AFTERNOON SNACK   2% milk-fat cottage cheese (¼ cup)

DINNER   Baked Lamb Shanks (4 ounces) with New
Potatoes* (2)
Sliced Raw Tomatoes with Dill and Lemon*
(½ cup)
Greek Fruit Salad* (½ cup)
Decaffeinated coffee, herb tea, mineral
water

EVENING SNACK   Plain low-fat yogurt (1 cup)

GREEK MENU

DAY 5

BREAKFAST I Unsweetened pineapple (½ cup)
2% milk-fat cottage cheese (¼ cup)
Whole-grain bread (1 slice)
Decaffeinated coffee, herb tea

OR

BREAKFAST II Banana (½)
Skim milk (1 cup)
Bran cereal (½ cup)
Decaffeinated coffee, herb tea

LUNCH Shrimp and Tomato Salad* (2 ounces
shrimp, ½ cup tomatoes)
Whole-wheat pita bread (1 slice)
Orange (1)
Decaffeinated coffee, herb tea, mineral
water

**AFTERNOON
SNACK** Apple (1)

DINNER Stuffed Eggplant* (1)
Cucumber and Yogurt Salad* (½ cup)
Spanish melon (⅛)
Decaffeinated coffee, herb tea, mineral
water

**EVENING
SNACK** Skim milk (1 cup)

GREEK MENU

BREAKFAST I   Unsweetened pineapple (½ cup)
2% milk-fat cottage cheese (¼ cup)
Whole-grain bread (1 slice)
Decaffeinated coffee, herb tea

OR

BREAKFAST II   Banana (½)
Skim milk (1 cup)
Bran cereal (½ cup)
Decaffeinated coffee, herb tea

LUNCH   Veal Kebabs* (1 patty)
Greek Salad II* (½ cup total vegetables)
Whole-wheat pita bread (1 slice)
Cantaloupe (¼)
Decaffeinated coffee, herb tea, mineral
water

AFTERNOON SNACK   2% milk-fat cottage cheese (¼ cup)

DINNER   Fish Plaki* (4 ounces)
Saffron Rice* (½ cup)
Steamed Zucchini with Dill and Lemon*
(½ cup)
Orange (1)
Decaffeinated coffee, herb tea, mineral
water

EVENING SNACK   Plain low-fat yogurt (1 cup)

187

GREEK MENU

BREAKFAST I   Unsweetened pineapple (½ cup)
2% milk-fat cottage cheese (¼ cup)
Whole-grain bread (1 slice)
Decaffeinated coffee, herb tea

OR

BREAKFAST II   Banana (½)
Skim milk (1 cup)
Bran cereal (½ cup)
Decaffeinated coffee, herb tea

LUNCH   Dolmitas* (Stuffed Grape Leaves) (4)
Greek Salad II* (½ cup total vegetables)
Grapefruit (½)
Decaffeinated coffee, herb tea, mineral
    water

AFTERNOON SNACK   Orange (1)

DINNER   Chilled Cucumber-Yogurt Soup* (1 cup)
Greek-Style Chicken* (4 ounces)
Saffron Rice* (½ cup)
Greek Salad III* (unlimited)
Fresh fig (1)
Decaffeinated coffee, herb tea, mineral
    water

EVENING SNACK   Skim milk (1 cup)

Mexican Menu

MEXICAN CUISINE HAS UNDERGONE many transformations over the centuries, and today the best-known and ever more popular Mexican food in the United States consists of the simple peasant staples. These are the tortillas, tacos, enchiladas and quesadillas, with their tasty fillings and sauces, all of which are adapted here to Southampton Diet specifications.

I highly recommend the Veracruz-style fish recipe with its interesting lime marinade. Serve it sizzling hot and you may feel yourself transported to the coast at Veracruz hearing the ocean surf in the background.

SHOPPING TIPS

• *Tortilla:* This is a flat pancake made from cornmeal. Tortillas form the basis for most of the recipes here and are available in the chilled dairy section of most supermarkets. They are excellent and easy to prepare. Muenster may be used in place of Monterey Jack cheese if the latter is not available.

• *Chile (or chile pepper):* A hot pepper of which there are many varieties, such as Jalapeño, a smooth one, from mid to dark green in color. The most characteristic seasoning of Mexican cuisine, chiles can be purchased either fresh or dried. But beware—they can be unpredictable! (See Cooking Tips below.)

• *Chayote:* Chayote, which is also called "vegetable pear," resembles a squash or gourd in appearance, and is thought to be indigenous to Mexico. It can be found in most large supermarkets on both coasts and in Spanish-American and West Indian markets in metropolitan areas. The chayote available in the United States nearly all year round is pale green to white in color and weighs about one pound. Since the vegetable has little taste and is watery, it needs to be dressed up with seasonings and sometimes cheese.

COOKING TIPS

• *Chile:* Sample all chiles before you use them, since, as I said, they are unpredictable. Do not touch your lips or eyes while you are preparing them. If you have sensitive skin, wear rubber gloves.

• *Taco:* A tortilla that is filled with shredded chicken, meat or cheese and shredded lettuce, tomatoes (and onions), is sometimes doused with sauce and then rolled up. The tacos commonly known in this country are fried in oil and filled with the same ingredients, but on this diet, they are prepared differently.

• *Quesadilla:* A tortilla that is filled with chicken, meat or cheese (or a combination of these ingredients) and folded in half and heated through.

• *Enchilada:* A tortilla that is filled with diced or shredded chicken or meat and cheese and onion, dipped in a sauce and rolled up. It is then covered with more of the same sauce and baked.

• *Salsa, or sauce:* Should be spiced according to your taste. Sauces may be hot in some households, relish-like in others. If the recipe calls for a food processor or blender, turn it on and off rapidly just to chop the ingredients.

MEXICAN MENU

BREAKFAST I Unsweetened pineapple (½ cup)
2% milk-fat cottage cheese (¼ cup)
Whole-grain bread (1 slice)
Decaffeinated coffee, herb tea

OR

BREAKFAST II Banana (½)
Skim milk (1 cup)
Bran cereal (½ cup)
Decaffeinated coffee, herb tea

LUNCH Turkey Taco* (1)
Ensalada I* (Mexican Salad) (unlimited)
Mango (½)
Decaffeinated coffee, herb tea, mineral
water

AFTERNOON SNACK Turkey breast* (1 ounce)

DINNER Chicken Breasts Picante con Chiles* (Spicy
Chicken Breasts with Chiles) (4 ounces)
Mexican Rice* (½ cup)
Ensalada II* (Mexican Salad) (½ cup total
vegetables)
Papaya (¾ cup)
Decaffeinated coffee, herb tea, mineral
water

EVENING SNACK Plain low-fat yogurt (1 cup)

MEXICAN MENU

DAY 2

BREAKFAST I Unsweetened pineapple (½ cup)
2% milk-fat cottage cheese (¼ cup)
Whole-grain bread (1 slice)
Decaffeinated coffee, herb tea

OR

BREAKFAST II Banana (½)
Skim milk (1 cup)
Bran cereal (½ cup)
Decaffeinated coffee, herb tea

LUNCH Ensalada III* (Mexican Salad) with Tuna
(½ cup tuna, ½ cup total chopped
vegetables)
Tortilla (1)
Orange (1)
Decaffeinated coffee, herb tea, mineral
water

AFTERNOON SNACK Plain low-fat yogurt (1 cup)

DINNER Veal Chops Veracruz* (4 ounces)
Mexican Rice* (½ cup)
Steamed Zucchini with Tomato Sauce*
(½ cup)
Ensalada I* (Mexican Salad) (unlimited)
Unsweetened diced pineapple (½ cup)
Decaffeinated coffee, herb tea, mineral
water

EVENING SNACK Banana (½)

MEXICAN MENU

BREAKFAST I Unsweetened pineapple (½ cup)
2% milk-fat cottage cheese (¼ cup)
Whole-grain bread (1 slice)
Decaffeinated coffee, herb tea

OR

BREAKFAST II Banana (½)
Skim milk (1 cup)
Bran cereal (½ cup)
Decaffeinated coffee, herb tea

LUNCH Monterey Jack Quesadilla* (1)
Ensalada I* (Mexican Salad) (unlimited)
Guava (1)
Decaffeinated coffee, herb tea, mineral
water

**AFTERNOON
SNACK** Tomato juice (½ cup)
Raw carrot sticks (½ cup)

DINNER Lime Chicken* (4 ounces)
Boiled corn on the cob (1 small ear) with
lime (garnish)
Ensalada II* (Mexican Salad) (½ cup total
chopped vegetables)
Spanish melon (⅛)
Decaffeinated coffee, herb tea, mineral
water

**EVENING
SNACK** Skim milk (1 cup)

MEXICAN MENU

DAY 4

BREAKFAST I   Unsweetened pineapple (½ cup)
2% milk-fat cottage cheese (¼ cup)
Whole-grain bread (1 slice)
Decaffeinated coffee, herb tea

OR

BREAKFAST II   Banana (½)
Skim milk (1 cup)
Bran cereal (½ cup)
Decaffeinated coffee, herb tea

LUNCH   Monterey Jack Taco* (1)
Ensalada I* (Mexican Salad) (unlimited)
Peach (1)
Decaffeinated coffee, herb tea, mineral
water

AFTERNOON SNACK   2% milk-fat cottage cheese (¼ cup)

DINNER   Veal en Salsa (in Sauce)* (4 ounces)
Mexican Rice* (½ cup)
Steamed Chayote with Tomato Sauce*
(½ cup)
Ensalada I* (Mexican Salad) (unlimited)
Papaya (¾ cup)
Decaffeinated coffee, herb tea, mineral
water

EVENING SNACK   Plain low-fat yogurt (1 cup)

194

MEXICAN MENU

DAY 5

BREAKFAST I   Unsweetened pineapple (½ cup)
2% milk-fat cottage cheese (¼ cup)
Whole-grain bread (1 slice)
Decaffeinated coffee, herb tea

OR

BREAKFAST II   Banana (½)
Skim milk (1 cup)
Bran cereal (½ cup)
Decaffeinated coffee, herb tea

LUNCH   Ensalada III (Mexican Salad) with Turkey*
(2 ounces turkey, ½ cup total vegetables)
Tortilla (1)
Pink grapefruit (½)
Decaffeinated coffee, herb tea, mineral
water

AFTERNOON   Apple (1)
SNACK

DINNER   Chicken Enchiladas* (1)
Steamed Green Beans* (½ cup) (page 238)
Ensalada I* (Mexican Salad) (unlimited)
Casaba melon (⅛)
Decaffeinated coffee, herb tea, mineral
water

EVENING   Skim milk (1 cup)
SNACK

195

MEXICAN MENU

DAY 6

BREAKFAST I Unsweetened pineapple (½ cup)
2% milk-fat cottage cheese (¼ cup)
Whole-grain bread (1 slice)
Decaffeinated coffee, herb tea

OR

BREAKFAST II Banana (½)
Skim milk (1 cup)
Bran cereal (½ cup)
Decaffeinated coffee, herb tea

LUNCH Chicken Taco* (1)
Ensalada I* (Mexican Salad) (unlimited)
Mango (½)
Decaffeinated coffee, herb tea, mineral
water

AFTERNOON SNACK 2% milk-fat cottage cheese (¼ cup)

DINNER Red Snapper Veracruz* (4 ounces)
Mexican Rice* (½ cup)
Steamed Cauliflower* (½ cup) (page 238)
Ensalada I* (Mexican Salad) (unlimited)
Strawberries (¾ cup)
Decaffeinated coffee, herb tea, mineral
water

EVENING SNACK Plain low-fat yogurt (1 cup)

196

MEXICAN MENU

BREAKFAST I   Unsweetened pineapple (½ cup)
2% milk-fat cottage cheese (¼ cup)
Whole-grain bread (1 slice)
Decaffeinated coffee, herb tea

OR

BREAKFAST II   Banana (½)
Skim milk (1 cup)
Bran cereal (½ cup)
Decaffeinated coffee, herb tea

LUNCH   Turkey and Monterey Jack Quesadilla* (1)
Ensalada I* (Mexican Salad) (unlimited)
Watermelon cubes (½ cup)
Decaffeinated coffee, herb tea, mineral
water

AFTERNOON SNACK   Orange (1)

DINNER   Pompano en Salsa Verde (in Green Tomato
Sauce)* (4 ounces)
Mexican Rice* (½ cup)
Steamed Summer Squash* (½ cup) (page
238)
Ensalada I* (Mexican Salad) (unlimited)
Sliced pineapple and banana (½ cup)
Decaffeinated coffee, herb tea, mineral
water

EVENING SNACK   Skim milk (1 cup)

197

Jewish Menu

THE JEWISH FOOD OF THE NEW YORK AREA has been celebrated by writers—including song writers—for at least a century. Delicatessens, where such food is served, are meeting places for all manner of celebrities, from stand-up comics to famous film and stage stars. Often these creative personalities not only head directly for their favorite establishments whenever they arrive in Manhattan, but rhapsodize about these "deli" dishes when they are out of town.

The food in these bustling restaurants has never, to my knowledge, been described as either light or delicate. One might logically assume that such fare would be far out of bounds for any dieter. For many of my patients, however, the total absence of these homey dishes would be perceived as a major psychological loss. As a result, I have gone to some pains to retrieve as many of these specialties as possible and to recast them to conform with the Southampton program.

If you are a deli lover, you will be surprised to find many of these hearty dishes here. Gefilte Fish, for instance, or Stuffed Cabbage Rolls or Borscht—yes, *with* the boiled potato. If you have never tasted this food, you might begin here on a new gastronomical adventure.

The ingredients can usually be found in any supermarket. The recipes are not difficult. A few, such as the Gefilte Fish or Stuffed Cabbage Rolls, require some time and effort, but over the years many traditional Jewish cooks have found them well worth the extra work.

I'm sure you will, too.

JEWISH MENU

DAY 1

BREAKFAST I   Unsweetened pineapple (½ cup)
2% milk-fat cottage cheese (¼ cup)
Whole-grain bread (1 slice)
Decaffeinated coffee, herb tea

OR

BREAKFAST II   Banana (½)
Skim milk (1 cup)
Bran cereal (½ cup)
Decaffeinated coffee, herb tea

LUNCH   *Salad plate of:* salmon (½ cup, canned),
sliced tomato (½ cup), raw onion slice,
cucumber and bed of lettuce (unlimited),
lemon wedge
Matzoh (half a 4″ x 6″ slice)
Grapefruit (½)
Decaffeinated coffee, herb tea, seltzer

AFTERNOON SNACK   Turkey breast* (1 ounce)

DINNER   Turkey Cutlets with Cranberry-Fruit Relish*
(4 ounces turkey, ½ cup relish)
Baked potato (1 small)
Steamed Carrots* (½ cup) (page 238)
Coleslaw Salad* (½ cup)
Decaffeinated seltzer

EVENING SNACK   Plain low-fat yogurt (1 cup)

199

JEWISH MENU

DAY 2

BREAKFAST I Unsweetened pineapple (½ cup)
2% milk-fat cottage cheese (¼ cup)
Whole-grain bread (1 slice)
Decaffeinated coffee, herb tea

OR

BREAKFAST II Banana (½)
Skim milk (1 cup)
Bran cereal (½ cup)
Decaffeinated coffee, herb tea

LUNCH *Open-face turkey sandwich of:* sliced Cooked
Turkey Breast* (page 237) (2 ounces),
sliced tomato (½ cup), lettuce (unlimited),
rye bread (1 slice)
Sliced peach (1)
Decaffeinated coffee, herb tea, seltzer

**AFTERNOON
SNACK** Plain low-fat yogurt (1 cup)

DINNER Stuffed Veal Rib Chops* (4 ounces)
Kasha (Buckwheat Groats)* (½ cup)
Cucumber Salad* (unlimited)
Baked Apple* (1)
Decaffeinated coffee, herb tea, seltzer

**EVENING
SNACK** Banana (½)

JEWISH MENU

DAY 3

BREAKFAST I
Unsweetened pineapple (½ cup)
2% milk-fat cottage cheese (¼ cup)
Whole-grain bread (1 slice)
Decaffeinated coffee, herb tea

OR

BREAKFAST II
Banana (½)
Skim milk (1 cup)
Bran cereal (½ cup)
Decaffeinated coffee, herb tea

LUNCH
Gefilte Fish* (2 ounces)
Salad plate of: sliced tomato (½ cup), sliced
cucumber (unlimited), bed of lettuce
(unlimited)
Matzoh (half a 4" x 6" slice)
Honeydew melon (⅛)
Decaffeinated coffee, herb tea, seltzer

AFTERNOON SNACK
Tomato juice (½ cup)
Raw carrot sticks (½ cup)

DINNER
Turkey Loaf* (4 ounces)
Baked potato (1 small)
Cold Pickled Beets* (½ cup)
Unsweetened Applesauce* (½ cup)
Decaffeinated coffee, herb tea, seltzer

EVENING SNACK
Skim milk (1 cup)

201

JEWISH MENU

DAY 4

BREAKFAST I
Unsweetened pineapple (½ cup)
2% milk-fat cottage cheese (¼ cup)
Whole-grain bread (1 slice)
Decaffeinated coffee, herb tea

OR

BREAKFAST II
Banana (½)
Skim milk (1 cup)
Bran cereal (½ cup)
Decaffeinated coffee, herb tea

LUNCH
Open-face sandwich of: sliced cold Turkey
Loaf* (2 ounces), lettuce (unlimited), rye
bread (1 slice)
Coleslaw Salad* (½ cup)
Cantaloupe (¼)
Decaffeinated coffee, herb tea, seltzer

AFTERNOON SNACK
2% milk-fat cottage cheese (¼ cup)

DINNER
Stuffed Cabbage Rolls* (2 rolls)
Steamed Carrots with Dill and Lemon*
(½ cup) (pages 238 and 304)
Cold Pickled Beets* (½ cup)
Unsweetened pineapple (½ cup)
Decaffeinated coffee, herb tea, seltzer

EVENING SNACK
Plain low-fat yogurt (1 cup)

JEWISH MENU

DAY 5

BREAKFAST I Unsweetened pineapple (½ cup)
2% milk-fat cottage cheese (¼ cup)
Whole-grain bread (1 slice)
Decaffeinated coffee, herb tea

OR

BREAKFAST II Banana (½)
Skim milk (1 cup)
Bran cereal (½ cup)
Decaffeinated coffee, herb tea

LUNCH Borscht* (1 cup, with 1 boiled potato)
Vegetables with farmer cheese (2 ounces
farmer cheese, ½ cup total chopped raw
tomato, carrot and celery)
Orange (1)
Decaffeinated coffee, herb tea, seltzer

AFTERNOON SNACK Apple (1)

DINNER Chicken in a Pot* (4 ounces chicken, ½ cup
cooked noodles, ½ cup carrots, 1 cup
broth)
Cucumber Salad* (unlimited)
Cantaloupe (¼)
Decaffeinated coffee, herb tea, seltzer

EVENING SNACK Skim milk (1 cup)

JEWISH MENU

DAY 6

BREAKFAST I   Unsweetened pineapple (½ cup)
2% milk-fat cottage cheese (¼ cup)
Whole-grain bread (1 slice)
Decaffeinated coffee, herb tea

OR

BREAKFAST II   Banana (½)
Skim milk (1 cup)
Bran cereal (½ cup)
Decaffeinated coffee, herb tea

LUNCH   *Open-face sandwich of:* Chopped Chicken
Liver* (2 ounces), sliced tomato (½ cup),
sliced cucumber (unlimited), lettuce
(unlimited), rye bread (1 slice)
Unsweetened Applesauce* (½ cup)
Decaffeinated coffee, herb tea, seltzer

AFTERNOON SNACK   2% milk-fat cottage cheese (¼ cup)

DINNER   Baked Fish with Tomato Sauce* (4 ounces)
Boiled noodles (½ cup)
Coleslaw Salad* (½ cup)
Broiled grapefruit (½)
Decaffeinated coffee, herb tea, seltzer

EVENING SNACK   Plain low-fat yogurt (1 cup)

JEWISH MENU

BREAKFAST I   Unsweetened pineapple (½ cup)
2% milk-fat cottage cheese (¼ cup)
Whole-grain bread (1 slice)
Decaffeinated coffee, herb tea

OR

BREAKFAST II   Banana (½)
Skim milk (1 cup)
Bran cereal (½ cup)
Decaffeinated coffee, herb tea

LUNCH   *Open-face sandwich of*: sliced smoked
salmon (2 ounces), sliced tomato (¼ cup),
raw onion slices (¼ cup), lettuce
(unlimited), bagel (½)
Pear (1)
Decaffeinated coffee, herb tea, seltzer

AFTERNOON SNACK   Plain low-fat yogurt (1 cup)

DINNER   Stuffed Peppers* (1)
Steamed Carrots with Dill and Lemon*
(½ cup) (pages 238 and 304)
Cucumber Salad* (unlimited)
Baked Apple* (1)
Decaffeinated coffee, herb tea, seltzer

EVENING SNACK   Skim milk (1 cup)

The Southampton Maintenance Diet

CONGRATULATIONS!

Reaching this point in the diet means that you have successfully shed all that unwanted weight. You have also experienced the pleasure of eating in a healthy, balanced manner. Your palate has been cleansed and refreshed and you have learned to eat in a way that brings you joy and the rewards of being slim.

Furthermore, because of the special balance of amino acids, carbohydrates and vitamins, you have achieved this new slenderness without the mood swings that so often accompany weight loss.

The Southampton Maintenance Diet that follows is a guideline for remaining thin and happy for the rest of your life. Since you require no further weight loss, certain foods not scheduled on Week 1 and 2 of the Southampton Diet can now be eaten in limited quantities. There are additional snacks, and the amounts of some foods have been increased for men.

The basic eating principles you have acquired, however, should not be forgotten. Planning out the food you will eat each day is one of those principles. Drawing most of your sustenance from the "happy" foods listed in Chapter 5 is another. And the psychological guidelines for controlling weight gain you have learned are, of course, equally important. All of these will protect you from regaining any portion of the weight you have lost.

The Maintenance Diet includes two plans—one for women and one for men. This distinction is based on the genetic differences in size and metabolic needs. In both cases, portion sizes have been increased and a small quantity of fat has been added.

A different breakfast is offered every day to give you more variety. Morning snacks have been added (after breakfast), and there are recipes for tasty fresh-fruit yogurt and skim-milk shakes and yogurt freezes. Butter (or margarine may be substituted, if desired) can be used on bread and sometimes on vegetables. Where a salad dressing is listed on the menu, simply use any of the dressing recipes in the Ethnic Diets section and add the appropriate amount of vegetable oil that is called for. I recommend polyunsaturated vegetable oil. Safflower oil is preferred, but corn or sunflower oils are also acceptable. The amount of dry white wine you can drink has been increased to four 4-ounce glasses or 16 ounces of wine a week.

You may follow this suggested plan for the Maintenance Diet which is simple and uses only a few recipes from the first chapter of the recipes section ("The Southampton Diet Recipes"). Or you may use any of the menus and recipes in the Ethnic Diets sections—simply increase the portions as listed here and add the extra fat or oil prescribed on the appropriate day's diet. Again, dishes with an asterisk (*) may be found in recipes section. No matter which menu you follow, I heartily recommend them to you for a lifetime of remaining Southampton thin and happy.

For your convenience, here is a listing of the breakfasts (there's a different one each day) and the snacks included in the Maintenance Diet for Women and Men. (Note that the men have the same breakfasts, but their portions have been increased or they have whole milk rather than skim milk.)

BREAKFASTS

	Women	Men
DAY 1	Unsweetened pineapple (½ cup)	(1 cup)
	2% milk-fat cottage cheese (¼ cup)	(¼ cup)
	Whole-grain bread (1 slice) with	(2 slices)
	butter (1 teaspoon)	(2 teaspoons)
	Decaffeinated coffee, herb tea	
DAY 2	Blueberries (½ cup)	(1 cup)
	Bran cereal (½ cup)	(1 cup)
	Skim milk (1 cup)	Whole milk (1 cup)
	Decaffeinated coffee, herb tea	
DAY 3	Grapefruit (½)	(1)
	Farmer cheese (¼ cup)	(¼ cup)
	Bran bread (1 slice) with butter	(2 slices)
	(1 teaspoon)	(2 teaspoons)
	Decaffeinated coffee, herb tea	
DAY 4	Fresh orange juice (½ cup)	(1 cup)
	Poached egg (1)	(1)
	Whole-wheat toast (1 slice) with	(2 slices)
	butter (1 teaspoon)	(2 teaspoons)
	Decaffeinated coffee, herb tea	
DAY 5	Cantaloupe (¼)	(½)
	2% milk-fat cottage cheese (¼ cup)	(¼ cup)
	Bran bread (1 slice) with butter	(2 slices)
	(1 teaspoon)	(2 teaspoons)
	Decaffeinated coffee, herb tea	
DAY 6	Banana (½)	(1)
	Skim milk (1 cup)	Whole milk (1 cup)
	Bran cereal (½ cup)	(1 cup)
	Decaffeinated coffee, herb tea	
DAY 7	Honeydew melon (⅛)	(¼)
	Soft-boiled egg (1)	(1)
	Whole-wheat toast (1 slice) with	(2 slices)
	butter (1 teaspoon)	(2 teaspoons)
	Decaffeinated coffee, herb tea	

SNACKS

	Morning Snack	Afternoon Snack	Evening Snack
DAY 1	Plain low-fat yogurt (1 cup) Banana (½)	Turkey breast* (1 ounce)	Strawberry Yogurt Freeze* (½ cup strawberries, 1 cup plain low-fat yogurt)
DAY 2	Plain low-fat yogurt (1 cup) Sliced apple (1)	Plain low-fat yogurt (1 cup)	Banana Shake* (½ banana, 1 cup skim milk)
DAY 3	Plain low-fat yogurt (1 cup) Strawberries (¾ cup)	Tomato juice (½ cup) Raw carrot sticks (½ cup)	Raspberry Shake* (½ cup raspberries, 1 cup skim milk)
DAY 4	Plain low-fat yogurt (1 cup) Unsweetened pineapple cubes (½ cup)	2% milk-fat cottage cheese (¼ cup)	Blueberry Shake* (½ cup blueberries, 1 cup plain low-fat yogurt)
DAY 5	Plain low-fat yogurt (1 cup) Banana (½)	Apple (1)	Pineapple Shake* (½ cup pineapple, 1 cup skim milk)
DAY 6	Plain low-fat yogurt (1 cup) Unsweetened pineapple cubes (½ cup)	2% milk-fat cottage cheese (¼ cup)	Banana Yogurt Freeze* (½ banana, 1 cup plain low-fat yogurt)
DAY 7	Plain low-fat yogurt (1 cup) Strawberries (¾ cup)	Orange (1)	Mango Shake* (½ cup mango, 1 cup skim milk)

Wine—four 4-ounce glasses or 16 ounces dry white wine per week

MAINTENANCE DIET—WOMEN

DAY 1

BREAKFAST   Unsweetened pineapple (½ cup)
2% milk-fat cottage cheese (¼ cup)
Whole-grain bread (1 slice) with butter
(1 teaspoon)
Decaffeinated coffee, herb tea

MORNING
SNACK   Plain low-fat yogurt (1 cup)
Banana (½)

LUNCH   *Open-face sandwich of:* sliced Cooked
Turkey Breast* (4 ounces), sliced tomato
(½ cup), sliced cucumber (unlimited),
lettuce (unlimited), whole-wheat bread (1
slice)
Apple (1)
Decaffeinated coffee, herb tea, mineral
water

AFTERNOON
SNACK   Turkey breast* (1 ounce)

DINNER   Broiled veal chop (4 ounces)
Brown Rice* (½ cup)
Steamed Zucchini* (½ cup)
Mixed green salad (unlimited)
Dressing* (unlimited with 2 teaspoons
vegetable oil)
Pear (1)
Decaffeinated coffee, herb tea, mineral
water

EVENING
SNACK   Strawberry Yogurt Freeze* (½ cup fresh or
frozen unsweetened strawberries and
1 cup plain low-fat yogurt)

MAINTENANCE DIET—WOMEN

DAY 2

BREAKFAST Blueberries (½ cup)
Bran cereal (½ cup), Skim milk (1 cup)
Decaffeinated coffee, herb tea

MORNING SNACK Plain low-fat yogurt (1 cup)
Sliced apple (1)

LUNCH *Southampton Salad Bowl of:* sliced hard-cooked egg (1), julienned Swiss cheese (1 ounce), julienned Cooked Turkey Breast* (2 ounces), tomato wedges (½ cup), sliced green pepper (¼ cup), sliced cucumber (unlimited), and mixed salad greens (unlimited)
Dressing* (unlimited with 1 teaspoon vegetable oil)
Whole-wheat bread (1 slice)
Cantaloupe (¼)
Decaffeinated coffee, herb tea, mineral water

AFTERNOON SNACK Plain low-fat yogurt (1 cup)

DINNER Broiled Chicken Breast* (4 ounces)
Baked potato (1 small) with butter (1 tsp.)
Steamed Broccoli* (½ cup)
Mixed green salad (unlimited)
Dressing* (unlimited with 1 teaspoon vegetable oil)
Strawberries (¾ cup) with Yogurt Topping* (1 tbsp.)
Decaffeinated coffee, herb tea, mineral water

EVENING SNACK Banana Shake* (½ banana and 1 cup skim milk)

211

MAINTENANCE DIET—WOMEN

DAY 3

BREAKFAST Grapefruit (½)
Farmer cheese (¼ cup)
Bran bread (1 slice) with butter (1 teaspoon)
Decaffeinated coffee, herb tea

MORNING SNACK Plain low-fat yogurt (1 cup)
Strawberries (¾ cup)

LUNCH *Southampton Salad Bowl of:* tuna (1 cup, canned), sliced tomato (½ cup), raw onion slice, mixed salad greens (unlimited)
Dressing* (unlimited with 1 teaspoon vegetable oil)
Rye bread (1 slice)
Honeydew melon (⅛)
Decaffeinated coffee, herb tea, mineral water

AFTERNOON SNACK Tomato juice (½ cup)
Raw carrot sticks (½ cup)

DINNER Roasted turkey breast (4 ounces)
Brown Rice* (½ cup)
Steamed Summer Squash* (½ cup)
Mixed green salad (unlimited)
Dressing* (unlimited with 1 teaspoon vegetable oil)
Orange (1)
Decaffeinated coffee, herb tea, mineral water

EVENING SNACK Raspberry Shake* (½ cup fresh or frozen unsweetened raspberries and 1 cup skim milk)

MAINTENANCE DIET—WOMEN

DAY 4

BREAKFAST Freshly squeezed orange juice (½ cup)
Poached egg (1)
Whole-wheat toast (1 slice) with butter
(1 teaspoon)
Decaffeinated coffee, herb tea

MORNING SNACK Plain low-fat yogurt (1 cup)
Unsweetened pineapple cubes (½ cup)

LUNCH *Open-face sandwich of:* sliced Muenster
cheese (4 ounces), sliced tomato (½ cup),
sliced cucumber (unlimited), romaine
lettuce (unlimited), whole-wheat bread
(1 slice)
Grapefruit (½)
Decaffeinated coffee, herb tea, mineral
water

AFTERNOON SNACK 2% milk-fat cottage cheese (¼ cup)

DINNER Baked Fish* (4 ounces)
Baked potato (1 small) with butter (1 tsp.)
Steamed Carrots* (½ cup)
Mixed green salad (unlimited)
Dressing* (unlimited with 1 teaspoon
vegetable oil)
Peach (1)
Decaffeinated coffee, herb tea, mineral
water

EVENING SNACK Blueberry Shake* (½ cup fresh or frozen
unsweetened blueberries and 1 cup plain
low-fat yogurt)

MAINTENANCE DIET—WOMEN

DAY 5

BREAKFAST   Cantaloupe (¼)
2% milk-fat cottage cheese (¼ cup)
Bran bread (1 slice) with butter (1 teaspoon)
Decaffeinated coffee, herb tea

MORNING   Plain low-fat yogurt (1 cup)
SNACK   Banana (½)

LUNCH   *Southampton Salad Bowl of:* julienned
Cooked Turkey Breast* (2 ounces),
julienned Swiss cheese (2 ounces), tomato
wedges (½ cup), sliced cucumber and
mixed salad greens (unlimited)
Dressing* (unlimited with 1 teaspoon
vegetable oil)
Whole-wheat bread (1 slice)
Pear (1)
Decaffeinated coffee, herb tea, mineral
water

AFTERNOON   Apple (1)
SNACK

DINNER   Lean roast beef (4 ounces)
Baked potato (1 small) with butter (1 tsp.)
Steamed Brussels Sprouts* (½ cup)
Mixed green salad (unlimited)
Vegetable oil (½ teaspoon) and vinegar
dressing
Plums (2)
Decaffeinated coffee, herb tea, mineral
water

EVENING   Pineapple Shake* (½ cup fresh or canned
SNACK   unsweetened pineapple and 1 cup skim
milk)

MAINTENANCE DIET—WOMEN

DAY 6

BREAKFAST Banana (½)
Skim milk (1 cup), Bran cereal (½ cup)
Decaffeinated coffee, herb tea

MORNING Plain low-fat yogurt (1 cup)
SNACK Unsweetened pineapple cubes (½ cup)

LUNCH *Southampton Salad Bowl of:* salmon (1 cup,
canned), sliced tomato (¼ cup), sliced
green pepper (¼ cup), onion slice, sliced
cucumber (unlimited) and mixed salad
greens (unlimited)
Dressing* (unlimited with 1 teaspoon
vegetable oil)
Whole-wheat bread (1 slice)
Apricots (2)
Decaffeinated coffee, herb tea, mineral
water

AFTERNOON 2% milk-fat cottage cheese (¼ cup)
SNACK

DINNER Broiled Fish* (4 ounces)
Brown Rice* (½ cup)
Steamed String Beans* (½ cup) with butter
(1 teaspoon)
Mixed green salad (unlimited)
Dressing* (unlimited with 1 teaspoon
vegetable oil)
Pineapple Ice* (½ cup)
Decaffeinated coffee, herb tea, mineral
water

EVENING Banana Yogurt Freeze* (½ banana and
SNACK 1 cup plain low-fat yogurt)

215

MAINTENANCE DIET—WOMEN

DAY 7

BREAKFAST   Honeydew melon (⅛)
Soft-boiled egg (1)
Whole-wheat toast (1 slice) with butter
   (1 teaspoon)
Decaffeinated coffee, herb tea

MORNING   Plain low-fat yogurt (1 cup)
SNACK   Strawberries (¾ cup)

LUNCH   *Open-face sandwich of:* tuna (1 cup,
   canned), sliced tomato (½ cup), sliced
   cucumber (unlimited), Boston lettuce
   (unlimited) and rye bread (1 slice)
Cantaloupe (¼)
Decaffeinated coffee, herb tea, mineral
   water

AFTERNOON   Orange (1)
SNACK

DINNER   Baked Chicken Breast* (4 ounces)
Wild Rice* (½ cup)
Steamed Spinach* (½ cup) with butter
   (1 teaspoon)
Mixed green salad (unlimited)
Dressing* (unlimited with 1 teaspoon
   vegetable oil)
Nectarine (1)
Decaffeinated coffee, herb tea, mineral
   water

EVENING   Mango Shake* (½ cup mango and 1 cup
SNACK   skim milk)

MAINTENANCE DIET—MEN

BREAKFAST Unsweetened pineapple (1 cup)
2% milk-fat cottage cheese (¼ cup)
Whole-grain bread (2 slices) with butter
(2 teaspoons)
Decaffeinated coffee, herb tea

MORNING SNACK Plain low-fat yogurt (1 cup)
Banana (½)

LUNCH *Sandwich of:* sliced Cooked Turkey Breast*
(4 ounces), sliced tomato (½ cup), sliced
cucumber (unlimited), lettuce
(unlimited), whole-wheat bread (2 slices)
Apple (1)
Decaffeinated coffee, herb tea, mineral
water

AFTERNOON SNACK Turkey breast* (1 ounce)

DINNER Broiled veal chop (6 ounces)
Brown Rice* (1 cup) with butter
(1 teaspoon)
Steamed Zucchini* (½ cup) with butter
(1 teaspoon)
Mixed green salad (unlimited)
Dressing* (unlimited with 2 teaspoons
vegetable oil)
Pear (1)
Decaffeinated coffee, herb tea, mineral
water

EVENING SNACK Strawberry Yogurt Freeze* (½ cup fresh or
frozen unsweetened strawberries and
1 cup plain low-fat yogurt)

MAINTENANCE DIET—MEN

DAY 2

BREAKFAST   Blueberries (1 cup)
Bran cereal (1 cup), Whole milk (1 cup)
Decaffeinated coffee, herb tea

**MORNING
SNACK**   Plain low-fat yogurt (1 cup)
Sliced apple (1)

LUNCH   *Southampton Salad Bowl of:* sliced hard-
cooked egg (1), julienned Swiss cheese
(1 ounce), julienned Cooked Turkey
Breast* (2 ounces), tomato wedges
(¼ cup), sliced green pepper (¼ cup),
sliced cucumber (unlimited), mixed salad
greens (unlimited)
Dressing* (unlimited with 2 teaspoons
vegetable oil)
Cantaloupe (¼)
Decaffeinated coffee, herb tea, mineral
water

**AFTERNOON
SNACK**   Plain low-fat yogurt (1 cup)

DINNER   Broiled Chicken Breast* (6 ounces)
Baked potato (1 small) with butter (1 tsp.)
Steamed Broccoli* (½ cup)
Mixed green salad (unlimited)
Dressing* (unlimited with 1 tsp. vegetable
oil)
Strawberries (¾ cup) with Yogurt Topping*
(1 tablespoon)
Decaffeinated coffee, herb tea, mineral
water

**EVENING
SNACK**   Banana Shake* (½ banana and 1 cup skim
milk)

218

MAINTENANCE DIET—MEN

DAY 3

BREAKFAST Grapefruit (1)
Farmer cheese (¼ cup)
Bran bread (2 slices) with butter (2 tsps.)
Decaffeinated coffee, herb tea

MORNING SNACK Plain low-fat yogurt (1 cup)
Strawberries (¾ cup)

LUNCH *Southampton Salad Bowl of:* tuna (1 cup, canned), sliced tomato (½ cup), raw onion slice, mixed salad greens (unlimited)
Dressing* (unlimited with 2 teaspoons vegetable oil)
Rye bread (2 slices)
Honeydew melon (⅛)
Decaffeinated coffee, herb tea, mineral water

AFTERNOON SNACK Tomato juice (½ cup)
Raw carrot sticks (½ cup)

DINNER Roasted turkey breast (6 ounces)
Brown Rice* (1 cup)
Steamed Summer Squash* (½ cup) with butter (1 teaspoon)
Mixed green salad (unlimited)
Dressing* (unlimited with 1 tsp. vegetable oil)
Orange (1)
Decaffeinated coffee, herb tea, mineral water

EVENING SNACK Raspberry Shake* (½ cup fresh or frozen unsweetened raspberries and 1 cup skim milk)

219

MAINTENANCE DIET—MEN

DAY 4

BREAKFAST Freshly squeezed orange juice (½ cup)
Poached egg (1)
Whole-wheat toast
(2 slices) with butter (2 teaspoons)
Decaffeinated coffee, herb tea

MORNING SNACK Plain low-fat yogurt (1 cup)
Unsweetened pineapple cubes (½ cup)

LUNCH *Sandwich of:* sliced Muenster cheese
(4 ounces), sliced tomato (½ cup), sliced
cucumber (unlimited), romaine lettuce
(unlimited), whole-wheat bread (2 slices)
Grapefruit (½)
Decaffeinated coffee, herb tea, mineral
water

AFTERNOON SNACK 2% milk-fat cottage cheese (¼ cup)

DINNER Baked Fish* (6 ounces)
Baked potato (1 small) with butter (1 tsp.)
Steamed Carrots* (½ cup) with butter
(1 teaspoon)
Mixed green salad (unlimited)
Dressing* (unlimited with 2 teaspoons
vegetable oil)
Peach (1)
Decaffeinated coffee, herb tea, mineral
water

EVENING SNACK Blueberry Shake* (½ cup fresh or frozen
unsweetened blueberries and 1 cup plain
low-fat yogurt)

MAINTENANCE DIET—MEN

DAY 5

BREAKFAST Cantaloupe (½)
2% milk-fat cottage cheese (¼ cup)
Bran bread (2 slices) with butter
(2 teaspoons)
Decaffeinated coffee, herb tea

MORNING SNACK Plain low-fat yogurt (1 cup)
Banana (½)

LUNCH *Southampton Salad Bowl of:* julienned
Cooked Turkey Breast* (2 ounces),
julienned Swiss cheese (2 ounces), tomato
wedges (½ cup), sliced cucumber
(unlimited), mixed salad greens
(unlimited)
Dressing* (unlimited with 2 teaspoons
vegetable oil)
Whole-wheat bread (2 slices)
Pear (1)
Decaffeinated coffee, herb tea, mineral
water

AFTERNOON SNACK Apple (1)

DINNER Lean roast beef (6 ounces)
Baked potato (1 small) with butter (1 tsp.)
Steamed Brussels Sprouts* (½ cup)
Mixed green salad (unlimited)
Vegetable oil (1 tsp.) and vinegar dressing
Plums (2)
Decaffeinated coffee, herb tea, mineral
water

EVENING SNACK Pineapple Shake* (½ cup unsweetened
pineapple and 1 cup skim milk)

MAINTENANCE DIET—MEN

DAY 6

BREAKFAST Banana (1)
Whole milk (1 cup)
Bran cereal (1 cup)
Decaffeinated coffee, herb tea

MORNING SNACK Plain low-fat yogurt (1 cup)
Unsweetened pineapple cubes (½ cup)

LUNCH *Southampton Salad Bowl of*: salmon (1 cup, canned), sliced tomato (¼ cup), sliced green pepper (¼ cup), onion slice, sliced cucumber and mixed salad greens (unlimited)
Dressing* (unlimited with 2 teaspoons vegetable oil)
Whole-wheat bread (2 slices)
Apricots (2)
Decaffeinated coffee, herb tea, mineral water

AFTERNOON SNACK 2% milk-fat cottage cheese (¼ cup)

DINNER Broiled Fish* (6 ounces)
Brown Rice* (1 cup) with butter (1 teaspoon)
Steamed String Beans* (½ cup)
Mixed green salad (unlimited)
Dressing* (unlimited with 1 teaspoon vegetable oil)
Pineapple Ice* (½ cup)
Decaffeinated coffee, herb tea, mineral water

EVENING SNACK Banana Yogurt Freeze* (½ banana and 1 cup plain low-fat yogurt)

MAINTENANCE DIET—MEN

DAY 7

BREAKFAST Honeydew melon (¼)
Soft-boiled egg (1)
Whole-wheat toast (2 slices) with butter
(2 teaspoons)
Decaffeinated coffee, herb tea

MORNING Plain low-fat yogurt (1 cup)
SNACK Strawberries (¾ cup)

LUNCH *Open-face sandwich of:* tuna (1 cup,
canned), sliced tomato (½ cup), sliced
cucumber (unlimited), Boston lettuce
(unlimited) and rye bread (2 slices)
Cantaloupe (¼)
Decaffeinated coffee, herb tea, mineral
water

AFTERNOON Orange (1)
SNACK

DINNER Baked Chicken Breast* (6 ounces)
Wild Rice* (1 cup)
Steamed Spinach* (½ cup) with butter
(2 teaspoons)
Mixed green salad (unlimited)
Dressing* (unlimited with 2 teaspoons
vegetable oil)
Nectarine (1)
Decaffeinated coffee, herb tea, mineral
water

EVENING Mango Shake* (½ cup mango and 1 cup
SNACK skim milk)

223

Questions and Answers

QUESTION: Does it matter if I skip a meal in the Southampton Diet?

ANSWER: Yes, indeed it does. For one thing, the diet is carefully balanced to provide for your body's nutritional needs, and skipping a meal would upset that balance. For another, the schedule of foods keeps you supplied with a proper level of glucose (sugar) as well as amino acids and the carbohydrates that assist them in reaching the brain. This balance helps you maintain the happy state of mind that is so important to dieting.

QUESTION: Does this apply to snacks as well?

ANSWER: Yes.

QUESTION: Why is breakfast exactly the same every day?

ANSWER: Because both the cottage cheese and/or yogurt in this meal contains tryptophan, the amino acid that will help you begin your day in a cheerful, well-balanced mood.

QUESTION: May I skip bread at breakfast and have it at lunch instead?

ANSWER: No. Bread is the source of the carbohydrate that helps tryptophan reach the brain.

QUESTION: Why does the Southampton Diet contain so much fish?

ANSWER: Because fish is low in saturated fats and cholesterol and therefore you can eat it in large quantities.

224

Although the question of the effects of cholesterol on the body is still a controversial one, I do not believe in infusing the body with excessive amounts of it. Since the body produces its own cholesterol, I see no reason to add to it unnecessarily through food.

QUESTION: *Why are veal and turkey provided in substantial quantities?*

ANSWER: Veal and turkey have high levels of tryptophan, but unlike beef and lamb, which also contain this "happy" amino acid, they are low in fat.

QUESTION: *May I add artificial sweeteners to my coffee or tea?*

ANSWER: Most artificial sweeteners do not affect the weight-loss process one way or the other, so you *can* use them, if necessary. I don't, however, recommend the use of *any* additives. This is part of the plan for a completely healthy diet. You may use lemon and/or skim milk, of course, but I do suggest that you attempt to wean yourself from using chemical sweeteners in your coffee or tea.

QUESTION: *Why should the coffee be decaffeinated and the tea herbal?*

ANSWER: Because the caffeine in regular coffee and tea is a stimulant to the central nervous system and can cause anxiety and depression. This effect works against the well-balanced state of mind created by the Southampton Diet. Caffeine is also potentially addictive. Switching to decaffeinated coffee and herbal tea will help you to feel relaxed and reduce anxiety.

QUESTION: *What kind of cottage cheese should I buy?*

ANSWER: Two percent low-fat cottage cheese is best. Regular cottage cheese is often "enriched" with milk products that contain fat.

QUESTION: *What bread is recommended?*

ANSWER: Whole-wheat breads that contain no additives or preservatives.

QUESTION: *Cereal is prescribed in the diet. What kind should I eat?*

ANSWER: Any cereal that has not been processed with additives or preservatives and is not coated with sugar. I especially recommend the natural bran cereals because of their high fiber content.

QUESTION: *What do I do if I get hungry between meals?*

ANSWER: On the Southampton Diet you will not be hungry between meals because, among other things, snacks are provided every two or three hours after every meal. If you do experience what you interpret as hunger, you should reread Chapter 7 on behavioral techniques and determine if, in fact, you are truly hungry or if what you are feeling is not simply a patterned response to some external stimulus.

QUESTION: *Can I eat as much of the mixed greens as I care to?*

ANSWER: Yes, you can, but bear in mind that your goal is to change your eating patterns and that excess eating of any kind—even when it does not interfere with weight loss—is discouraged.

QUESTION: *Are diet sodas included on the diet?*

ANSWER: Diet sodas contain chemical additives and are not, therefore, included on the Southampton Diet. I do not recommend them.

QUESTION: *What kind of milk can I drink?*

ANSWER: Skim milk or ninety-eight percent or ninety-nine percent fat-free milk is permitted.

QUESTION: *Do you recommend dietetic candies?*

ANSWER: No. You should have no need for them on the Southampton Diet.

QUESTION: *What about chewing gum?*

ANSWER: No. *All* gum stimulates gastric juices.

QUESTION: How much alcohol is allowed?

ANSWER: You may drink eight ounces of white wine per week. I suggest that you mix an ounce or two with soda to make a spritzer.

QUESTION: How much water should I drink?

ANSWER: As much as you like. Water cleanses the body, so the more the better. It can also give you a pleasant feeling of fullness.

QUESTION: Won't I retain all that water?

ANSWER: No. As long as you are healthy, you will not retain it.

QUESTION: What kind of nonstick pan should I use?

ANSWER: From my experience, Silverstone cookware has proved to be the best. The Silverstone nonstick surface now coats pans made of heavy-gauge aluminum and has an excellent, durable cooking surface. Just be certain to use plastic or wooden utensils on nonstick pans to prevent scratching.

QUESTION: If the food still sticks, should I add liquid?

ANSWER: Yes. Chicken or vegetable broth, water or tomato juice can be added to the pan.

QUESTION: What about nonstick sprays?

ANSWER: I don't recommend them because they have additives and impart a certain flavor that can change the taste of the food.

QUESTION: When should I weigh the food portions?

ANSWER: Weigh and measure all foods after cooking, at least for the first four days on the diet. After that, you will be able to estimate the weight by sight.

QUESTION: Do you recommend appetite suppressants, thyroid medications, water pills or diuretics?

227

ANSWER: There are absolutely no pills on the Southampton Diet. Any medications should be prescribed by your physician.

QUESTION: *Tryptophan is available in pills. Should I take these?*

ANSWER: No. The proper amount of tryptophan is regulated in the diet.

QUESTION: *How long can I stay on the South-ampton Diet?*

ANSWER: Indefinitely. After Week 1 of the diet, you can follow Week 2 or any of the Ethnic Diets for as long as you want.

QUESTION: *When should I weigh myself?*

ANSWER: Weigh yourself (nude) every four days before breakfast. Do not weigh yourself more often than this, because the weight change you notice from day to day may not be an accurate recording of real gains or losses.

QUESTION: *Why should I remove the skin from chicken?*

ANSWER: Because it contains a heavy layer of fat.

QUESTION: *Can I use instant broth or bouillon?*

ANSWER: For cooking purposes only, not for a snack.

QUESTION: *Should all the vegetables be fresh?*

ANSWER: Yes. If possible, use only fresh vegetables. They are highest in fiber, nutrient and vitamin content. If fresh vegetables are not available, you may substitute frozen ones.

QUESTION: *Is four ounces the same as one-half cup of food?*

ANSWER: No, not necessarily. Cups and ounces represent measurements of two different things: *volume* and *weight*. Liquids are usually measured by volume in containers such as cups, and solids are usually weighed on a scale.

228

QUESTION: Can salt be used to add flavor to foods?

ANSWER: It should only be used in cooking, not for seasoning already cooked foods. There is increasing evidence that excess salt contributes to cardiovascular disease. Also, sodium helps to retain fluids in the body.

QUESTION: Can wine vinegar be used in salad dressings?

ANSWER: Yes, it can.

QUESTION: When I'm dining in a restaurant and a salad already has dressing on it, should I eat it?

ANSWER: No. Learn to order a plain salad before this course comes to the table. If you forget, apologize to the waiter for your error in ordering and request a plain salad with vinegar or lemon.

QUESTION: What kind of herb tea should I drink?

ANSWER: Any variety, as long as it does not contain caffeine. Decaffeinated teas such as the orange pekoe variety are fine. The commercial tea companies are now producing herb teas, which can be found in most supermarkets. If not, the teas can always be purchased in health food stores.

QUESTION: What if a long period elapses between meals?

ANSWER: The Southampton Diet specifically provides snacks between meals. Being conscious of the timing of these prescribed snacks is important.

QUESTION: If fresh fruit is not available, what should I eat instead?

ANSWER: Only fruit that is packed in its own juice (with the juice drained), or frozen varieties without added sugar.

QUESTION: Can I use commercial dietetic salad dressing?

ANSWER: I don't recommend any of these. The

recipes for salad dressings appear in the recipes section of this book.

QUESTION: *How much salad dressing can I use?*

ANSWER: You can use as much as you want, because the recipes in this book are free of all oil.

QUESTION: *Can I switch lunch and dinner meals?*

ANSWER: No. You should follow the diet as prescribed. The diet has been planned with consideration of blood chemistry and its effect on appetite.

QUESTION: *Why is a carbohydrate included at every meal?*

ANSWER: To provide a mechanism for amino acids to reach the brain.

QUESTION: *Can I pan-fry a veal burger in a nonstick pan?*

ANSWER: No. All meat should be cooked on an open rack so that the fat is not reabsorbed.

QUESTION: *Why is fat permitted on the Maintenance Diet?*

ANSWER: Because the body requires certain fatty acids to be healthy. They are on the diet, in limited amounts, as butter for spreading on bread or vegetables or as safflower and corn oils in dressings.

QUESTION: *How should I order in a restaurant?*

ANSWER: Order the prescribed meal on the Southampton Diet with the meat or fish broiled, baked or poached, without any additional fat. Vegetables should not be cooked with butter or oil and none should be added. Ask the waiter to eliminate any sauces or gravies or push them to the side. Ask him to prepare the food specially to your order. If the portion is larger than specified on the diet, leave the extra amount on your plate.

QUESTION: *If I am invited to a friend's home for dinner, should I save my calories all day for the dinner?*

ANSWER: No. The Southampton Diet has been specially developed so that you can feel comfortable and happy while you lose weight. This unique effect on mood can only occur if you eat the portions prescribed on the diet at the proper intervals.

QUESTION: *What should I do if I'm going to a cocktail party?*

ANSWER: Familiarize yourself with the prescribed eating program for that day so that you can stay on the diet. The Southampton Diet provides an opportunity to drink wine as well as have a snack. If the cocktail party is a lengthy one, I suggest that you dilute your wine with soda water.

QUESTION: *Do you recommend fasting once a week?*

ANSWER: No. Fasting causes muscle wasting, vital organ destruction and mineral depletion. It also has severe effects on mood, causing depression and lethargy.

QUESTION: *Can I drink tonic water instead of club soda?*

ANSWER: No. Tonic has as much sugar as colas. Bitter Lemon also contains sugar.

QUESTION: *Is cream cheese allowed on the diet?*

ANSWER: No. Cream cheese contains high amounts of fat and few helpful amino acids.

QUESTION: *Do you suggest prune juice or dried fruits to combat constipation?*

ANSWER: You should not become constipated on the Southampton Diet. And I don't recommend prune juice or dried fruits in any case, because they contain high concentrations of sugar. If constipation is a problem, consult your physician.

QUESTION: *What kind of tuna fish should I buy?*

ANSWER: Most kinds packed in water.

QUESTION: *Why are canned tuna and salmon and cottage cheese measured in cups and not ounces?*

ANSWER: Because it is more exact to measure them in this form.

QUESTION: What fats are excluded from the Southampton Diet?

ANSWER: Almost all fats, including butter, margarine, cream cheese, sweet cream and sour cream, mayonnaise and any kind of oil. The only exception to this rule is when small amounts are called for in some recipes for seasoning the nonstick pan when cooking. To season a pan, dip a piece of paper towel in a small amount of oil (vegetable), about 1 teaspoon, and rub it around the inside of the pan.

QUESTION: Does this rule apply to diet margarine and mayonnaise?

ANSWER: Yes.

QUESTION: How do I maintain my weight once it is lost?

ANSWER: The Southampton Diet provides you with a maintenance diet. This is a liberal program that you can follow for the rest of your life. It will change your eating habits forever and you will have no trouble maintaining your new lower weight.

QUESTION: What are the guidelines for maintaining the weight that I have achieved?

ANSWER: Stay within the parameters of the Maintenance Diet. Weigh yourself once every four days. If you gain more than two pounds, resume the first week of the Southampton Diet until you reach two to three pounds below your ideal weight. Remember to weigh yourself at the same hour of the day each time.

QUESTION: Can fruit juices be interchanged with fruit?

ANSWER: Yes. Four ounces of fruit juice can be used in place of a piece of fruit. But remember that you will be giving up the chewing satisfaction and the fiber content necessary for good digestion.

QUESTION: Should I go on the Southampton Diet if I am pregnant?

ANSWER: *No!* The diet of a pregnant woman should be individually monitored by her obstetrician. There are many special nutritional considerations for the pregnant diet. You can begin the diet after delivery if you are not breast feeding.

QUESTION: *Should adolescents go on this diet?*

ANSWER: No. The nutritional needs of an adolescent are multifaceted and must be evaluated on an individual basis.

QUESTION: *Other than pregnant women and adolescents, is this diet recommended for everyone?*

ANSWER: It is recommended for everyone who is healthy. For those who have certain medical disorders (described in the Appendix), it is not. These disorders require the attention of a physician.

QUESTION: *Should I exercise while on this diet?*

ANSWER: A moderate plan of exercise is recommended. You should consult with your physician before undertaking any *strenuous* exercise program.

QUESTION: *Can I have blueberry yogurt instead of adding fresh blueberries to yogurt?*

ANSWER: No. Commercial brands of yogurt that contain fruit also contain substantial amounts of sugar. Mixing yogurt with the fruit from your evening meal will add a nice fruity flavor to your yogurt. Recipes for shakes and freezes are included on the Maintenance Diet.

QUESTION: *Why can't I eat one whole banana at one meal instead of half a banana at breakfast and half for a snack?*

ANSWER: It is important to maintain an equal distribution of carbohydrates at each meal.

QUESTION: *Why is yogurt so important?*

ANSWER: Because it is very high in tryptophan and also contains the culture lactobacillus, which provides a helpful medium to absorb B vitamins.

QUESTION: *When should I eat my snacks?*

ANSWER: Timing is important. Snacks should be eaten two to three hours after meals.

QUESTION: *Can I have my evening snack at dinnertime?*

ANSWER: No, but you can do something even better. You can save the fruit from dinner and use it in the yogurt or yogurt freeze or skim-milk shake. This is a delicious midevening snack, and you will find the recipes in the Maintenance diet recipe section of this book.

QUESTION: *What should I do if I miss a snack?*

ANSWER: Continue on the daily diet plan and eat the next meal. But try not to do this on a regular basis.

QUESTION: *Must I have the snacks every day, even when I don't feel hungry?*

ANSWER: Yes. It is important to eat the snacks as well as the three meals on the Southampton Diet in order to maintain carbohydrate and amino acid balance.

THE
RECIPES

The Southampton Diet Recipes

Cooked (Poached) Chicken or Turkey Breasts for Sandwiches, Salads or Snacks

4 ounces chicken or turkey breast, boned and skinned
Water or chicken stock to cover
1 carrot, halved
1 celery rib, halved
1 small onion, halved
5 sprigs parsley
5 sprigs dill
1 clove garlic, split
6 black peppercorns
Pinch of salt

1. Place chicken in a small saucepan Add water or chicken stock to cover and the rest of the ingredients.
2. Bring mixture to a boil and simmer, covered, for 15 to 20 minutes, turning the chicken once. Do not overcook. Remove from heat, strain the broth and refrigerate chicken and broth separately until needed. (The chicken broth can be used for any of the recipes that require it.) Discard the vegetables.

2 SERVINGS (1 SERVING = 2 OUNCES)

Brown Rice

DAYS 1, 3, 4 AND 6; WEEKS 1 AND 2

½ cup brown rice
1¾ cups water or stock (chicken, veal, beef, fish or
  vegetable to match the main course)
Pinch of salt, if desired

1. Wash the rice carefully in several changes of cool water to remove any particles (such as sand or discolored rice grains) that may surface.
2. Combine rice, water or stock and salt in a small saucepan.
3. Bring the mixture to a boil on high heat, uncovered, and immediately reduce to a low simmer. Shake pot (to loosen grains apart) and cover tightly.
4. Cook for approximately 40 minutes, turn off heat and let rice stand for another 10 minutes. Remove the lid. The rice should be tender but not mushy.
5. Separate the grains with a fork and serve immediately.

NOTE: Before cooking, you may also want to add ¾ teaspoon of curry powder and/or any other herb or spice for a more flavorful and exotic taste.

3 SERVINGS (1 SERVING = ½ CUP)

Steamed Fresh Vegetables

The most nutritious way to cook most vegetables is by steaming them. This can be accomplished by placing the vegetable on a stainless steel vegetable steamer and then into a deep pot with a cover. Use a pot that will not impart a metallic flavor

238

to the vegetables during the steaming process, such as stainless steel, glass or enamel, but preferably not aluminum.

1. Clean the vegetables well in water. Pour 1 to 2 inches of water into the pot, making certain that the water doesn't touch the bottom of the steamer. Dense, hard vegetables such as carrots, broccoli or cauliflower are best cut into smaller pieces to shorten the cooking time; soft vegetables such as zucchini or other squash should be left in larger pieces. A clove of garlic (slivered), sliced ginger root, dill or parsley or some dried herbs may be added for more flavor.

2. Cover the pan, bring water to a boil over medium-high heat and steam the vegetables until they are tender but still crisp. If a sharp knife can pierce the vegetable, it is done. Leaf vegetables such as spinach are cooked when they have wilted and are reduced to about one-half their uncooked amount. The cooking time is also contingent on the toughness, size and age of vegetable.

3. Remove from heat and, if desired, squeeze on fresh lemon juice and season with any additional herbs or spices.

NOTE: Fresh vegetables may also be boiled, baked whole (such as potatoes or beets) or sautéed quickly over high heat in vegetable or chicken stock in a nonstick pan, but precious vitamins and minerals may be lost during the cooking process. Also the Vegetables cookbook from The Good Cook series, published by Time-Life, is a fine reference if you want to find out the specific cooking times for every kind of vegetable.

Broiled Chicken Breast
DAY 2, WEEKS 1 AND 2

4 ounces chicken breast
4 tablespoons lemon or lime juice, tomato juice or
    chicken stock
½ clove garlic, smashed
1 teaspoon chopped fresh dill or parsley, and/or
    ¼ teaspoon each dried rosemary, oregano, basil,
    tarragon, thyme (or your favorite herb or herbs in any
    combination)
Salt, if desired, and freshly ground pepper to taste
½" chunk of fresh ginger root, thinly sliced, and/or
    ½–1 teaspoon Dijon mustard (optional)

1. Remove the skin from the chicken.
2. Mix together remaining ingredients in a bowl just large enough to hold the chicken. Add the chicken breast and turn to coat evenly. Let sit for 15 minutes (or longer if desired). Turn the chicken twice more during this time.
3. Place chicken and marinade in a nonstick pan or in a regular broiling pan lined with aluminum foil. Cook under broiler on meaty side first until chicken turns white, basting with the marinade, about 5 minutes. Turn the breast over, baste again and broil on underside for an additional 5 minutes or until meat is done. Serve immediately.

NOTE: The juice or stock can be used in combination: such as 2 tablespoons of lemon juice mixed with 2 tablespoons of chicken stock.

1 SERVING

Baked Fish

DAY 4, WEEKS 1 AND 2

*4 ounces of fresh fish fillets (i.e., sole, flounder, halibut,
scrod, trout, bluefish), or 4 ounces fresh fish steaks
(i.e., salmon, swordfish, tuna)*
*4 tablespoons lemon or lime juice, tomato juice, fish or
chicken stock*
½ clove garlic, smashed
*1 teaspoon chopped fresh parsley or dill, and/or
¼ teaspoon crushed dried herbs (basil, fennel, oregano,
rosemary or thyme)*
Salt, if desired, and freshly ground pepper to taste
½" chunk fresh ginger root, thinly sliced (optional)
Garnish: thin slices of lemon or lime

1. Preheat oven to 350° F.
2. Mix together all of the ingredients in a bowl just
large enough to hold the fish. Add the fish fillet or steak and turn
to coat evenly. Let sit for 15 minutes (or longer if desired), turning the fish once more.
3. Bake, uncovered, in a shallow nonstick pan until
just done—about 10 to 15 minutes depending on thickness of
fish, basting with the liquid. Add more if needed. The fish
should flake easily when tested with a fork. Do not overcook.
4. Serve immediately garnished with lemon or lime
slices.

NOTE: An even simpler method of cooking is to steam
fish in the oven by wrapping it in aluminum foil. This requires
no basting: After marinating, place the fish fillet or steak on sheet
of foil and spoon over marinade. Seal in foil and bake in 425° F.
preheated oven until done, about 10 to 15 minutes.

The juice or stock can be used in combination: such
as 2 tablespoons of lemon juice mixed with 2 tablespoons of fish
stock.

1 SERVING

Broiled Fish

DAY 6, WEEKS 1 and 2

Use the same ingredients and instructions as for Baked Fish except place the fish in a nonstick pan under a pre-heated broiler. Broil 2 inches away from heat for 5 to 10 minutes, basting with the marinade. If cooking fish steaks, turn fish on other side after it turns color—about 5 minutes—and cook until just done. (It is done when the fish flakes apart easily when tested with a fork.) Do not overcook. Serve immediately, garnished with lemon or lime slices.

1 SERVING

Baked Chicken Breast

DAY 7, WEEKS 1 and 2

4 ounces chicken breast
4 tablespoons lemon or lime juice, tomato juice or
*   chicken stock*
½ clove garlic, smashed
1 teaspoon chopped fresh dill or parsley
¼ teaspoon each dried rosemary, oregano, basil,
*   tarragon, thyme (or your favorite herb or herbs in any*
*   combination)*
Salt, if desired, and freshly ground pepper to taste
½" chunk of fresh ginger root, thinly sliced, and/or
*   ½–1 teaspoon Dijon mustard (optional)*

1. Preheat oven to 350° F.
2. Remove the skin from the chicken.
3. Mix together the remaining ingredients in a bowl just large enough to hold the chicken. Add the chicken breast

242

and turn to coat evenly. Let sit for 15 minutes (or longer if desired). Turn the chicken twice more during this time.

4. Place chicken and marinade in nonstick baking dish into the preheated oven. Bake, basting with the liquid (add more if needed) until done—about 10 to 15 minutes.

NOTE: An even simpler method of cooking is to steam chicken in the oven by wrapping the breast in aluminum foil. This requires no basting: After marinating, place the chicken on sheet of foil and spoon the marinade over it. Seal in the foil and bake in 425° F. preheated oven until done, about 10 to 15 minutes.

The juice or stock can also be used in combination: such as 2 tablespoons of lemon juice mixed with 2 tablespoons of chicken stock.

1 SERVING

Wild Rice

DAY 7, WEEKS 1 and 2

1 cup wild rice
4 cups water
Pinch of salt, if desired

1. Place the rice in a bowl and add cool water to cover. Remove any foreign particles that float to the top, and drain the rice in a colander. Repeat this same procedure.

2. Bring the water and salt to a boil. Stir the rice slowly into the boiling salted water. Cook it on medium heat without stirring until tender, about 40 minutes. Serve immediately.

4 SERVINGS (1 SERVING = ½ CUP)

French and Nouvelle Cuisine Recipes

Niçoise Salad

DAY 1

Romaine lettuce (unlimited quantity)
1 cup (7-ounce can) tuna (packed in water, drained)
⅓ cup cold string beans (steamed 5–8 minutes, see page 238)
⅓ cup tomato wedges
⅓ cup thinly sliced red or green pepper
2 tablespoons capers (optional)
Vinaigrette Dressing I or II

1. Arrange lettuce in a bowl. Place tuna (which has been flaked apart) in the center and surround with string beans (divided into 2 bundles), tomato wedges and sliced pepper. Sprinkle on capers, if desired.

2. Spoon on dressing and serve.

2 SERVINGS (1 SERVING = ½ CUP TUNA; ½ CUP TOTAL VEGETABLES)

Vinaigrette Dressing I

2 teaspoons Dijon mustard
5 tablespoons chicken stock
1 clove garlic, peeled and mashed
½ teaspoon minced fresh chervil or parsley, or
  ¼ teaspoon dried
2 leaves fresh basil, minced
1 tablespoon wine vinegar
1 tablespoon lemon juice
¼ teaspoon freshly ground pepper

Combine ingredients in screw-top jar, cover and shake well. Refrigerate until used. Remove garlic with spoon and shake again before serving.

YIELD: ½ CUP

Vinaigrette Dressing II

1 cup water
¼ cup white wine
2 teaspoons salt
¼ cup red wine vinegar or fresh lemon juice
½ teaspoon pepper
½ teaspoon dry mustard
½ teaspoon dried basil
¼ cup chopped parsley
1 clove garlic, finely chopped

Combine ingredients in screw-top jar, cover and shake well. Can be refrigerated until used. Shake again before serving.

YIELD: 1¾ CUPS

245

Poached Chicken Breasts Tarragon
DAYS 1 AND 2

3 (about 12 ounces) chicken breasts, skinned and boned
2–3 cups water and/or chicken stock (to cover)
1 rib celery, julienned
1 bay leaf
½ small onion, peeled and quartered
1 clove garlic, split
1 sprig parsley
1 carrot, peeled and julienned
4 peppercorns
¼ teaspoon salt
½ teaspoon dried tarragon
Garnish: watercress sprigs

1. Place chicken breasts in a saucepan.
2. Add water or stock, celery, bay leaf, onion, garlic, parsley, carrot, peppercorns, salt and tarragon to the saucepan and simmer 15 to 20 minutes until the breast meat is tender. Strain and reserve the liquid, chicken, carrot and celery.
3. To make sauce (Viande Glace), pour 1 cup of the chicken broth into saucepan and boil gently until only 4 tablespoons liquid remain. The sauce will be slightly thick and have a strong chicken flavor.
4. Arrange one chicken breast on each plate with the reserved julienned carrot and celery rib and garnish each with a sprig of watercress. Spoon sauce over chicken and vegetables.
5. Refrigerate leftover chicken breast overnight for lunch the following day. Serve it thinly sliced, garnished with a lemon wedge, tomato slice and watercress.

4 SERVINGS: 2 DINNER (4 OUNCES EACH) AND 2 LUNCH (2 OUNCES EACH)

Cauliflower Puree

DAY 1

1 cup cauliflower flowerettes
2 pinches of coarse salt
¼ cup skim milk (optional)
Pinch of grated nutmeg
Salt and freshly ground pepper

1. Place the cauliflower in a saucepan, add water to cover and the coarse salt. Bring to a boil and simmer until tender, about 20 minutes. Drain.
2. Add skim milk, if desired.
3. Puree mixture in electric blender or food processor. Reheat in double boiler. Add the nutmeg and salt and pepper to taste.

2 SERVINGS (1 SERVING = ½ CUP)

Sautéed Snow Peas with Shallots and Basil

DAY 2

2 cups fresh snow peas
1 cup chicken stock
2 tablespoons minced shallots
Salt and freshly ground pepper
2 teaspoons chopped fresh basil

1. Remove the stringlike fiber running along both sides of the snow peas and cut off the stem ends.
2. Steam the snow peas for 2 to 3 minutes in a vegetable steamer (see page 238) until they are tender but still crisp. Drain the water and set aside.
3. Place the chicken stock in a saucepan and heat

until it has reduced to about 4 tablespoons. Add the shallots and cook them slowly for 1 to 2 minutes until they are soft. Turn the heat to medium-high and sauté the snow peas, stirring constantly with a wooden spoon, for about 1 minute.

4. Season with salt and pepper to taste, sprinkle on the basil and serve.

4 SERVINGS (1 SERVING = ½ CUP)

Veal Pâté

DAYS 2 AND 3

1¼ *pounds lean ground veal*
1 *tablespoon cognac*
2 *teaspoons chopped shallots*
½ *teaspoon dried savory*
½ *teaspoon dried basil*
½ *teaspoon fresh chopped parsley*
4 *ounces tomato puree*
2 *egg whites*
¼ *teaspoon salt*
½ *teaspoon freshly ground pepper*
Garnish: 4 mushrooms

1. Preheat oven to 350° F.

2. Place all ingredients except the mushrooms in a large mixing bowl.

3. Beat them well for several minutes with a wooden spoon so that the mixture is light and airy. Mold into a nonstick loaf pan, and garnish with the mushrooms.

4. Bake for 1 to 1¼ hours until done. Pâté should have shrunk and juices run clear when tested. Remove from oven and let stand 10 minutes to set. Serve hot.

5. Refrigerate remaining loaf overnight. Serve cold, thinly sliced, the following day for lunch.

6 SERVINGS: 2 DINNER (4 OUNCES EACH) AND 4 LUNCH (2 OUNCES EACH)

Ratatouille
(Eggplant, Tomatoes and Zucchini)

DAYS 2 AND 3

1 *medium-size onion, chopped*
2–3 *plum tomatoes, peeled, seeded and chopped*
1 *medium-size eggplant, peeled and cubed*
3 *medium-size zucchini, peeled and sliced*
3 *red or green peppers, halved, seeded, deribbed and*
  cubed
1 *clove garlic, crushed*
1 *Bouquet Garni*
Salt and freshly ground pepper to taste

BOUQUET GARNI
Bouquet garni consists of 3 sprigs fresh chervil, 3 sprigs fresh parsley, 2 sprigs fresh thyme and ½ bay leaf tied in a bunch. If you cannot obtain fresh materials, wrap 1 teaspoon dried thyme, 1 bay leaf, 1 teaspoon dried chervil and 2 teaspoons fresh parsley in a small square of cheesecloth. Tie together with string.

1. Cook the onion carefully in a large, covered non-stick pan over low to medium heat for about 10 minutes until it is softened. (Since the onion smell may be very strong it may be wise to keep your kitchen fan going.) Add chicken broth or water if necessary.

2. Add the tomatoes and cook several more minutes. Then add the eggplant, zucchini, red or green peppers, garlic, Bouquet Garni, salt and pepper. Cover the pan. Simmer for 30 to 40 minutes over low heat, or until vegetables have softened and there is a substantial amount of liquid. Uncover and continue cooking slowly for 5 to 15 minutes more to reduce the liquid. Stir to prevent burning.

3. Serve hot.

4. Refrigerate remaining dish overnight and serve cold the following day for lunch.

6 SERVINGS (1 SERVING = ½ CUP)

Baked Salmon Mousse

DAY 3

1 tablespoon tomato puree
¼ cup skim milk
1 egg white
2 tablespoons fresh lemon juice, or juice of 1 large lemon
2 tablespoons nonfat dry milk powder
1½ cups fresh salmon, or 1 7-ounce can, drained
¼ cup fresh bread crumbs
½ medium-size onion, chopped
Salt and freshly ground pepper to taste
½ teaspoon fresh dill, or ¼ teaspoon dried
¼ cup chopped celery
½ cup chopped green pepper
1 cup Pureed Tomato Sauce (optional) (page 251)
Garnish: watercress

1. Preheat oven to 350° F.

2. Put all ingredients except celery and green pepper pieces into blender, with liquids at the bottom. Puree until smooth.

3. Scatter celery and green pepper into nonstick ring mold. Pour contents of blender into mold and bake for 40 minutes.

4. Unmold onto serving platter and garnish with watercress. Serve hot, or refrigerate and serve cold next day. If desired, the Pureed Tomato Sauce can accompany the salmon.

3 SERVINGS (1 SERVING = ⅔ CUP)

Pureed Tomato Sauce

DAY 3

2 cups chicken or veal stock
3 shallots, peeled and chopped
1 clove garlic, crushed
1 Bouquet Garni (page 249)
8 ounces tomato puree
Salt and freshly ground pepper

1. Heat ½ cup stock in a nonstick saucepan and cook shallots on low heat until transparent, about 8 minutes.
2. Add the rest of ingredients and simmer, covered, for 15 minutes.
3. Remove Bouquet Garni and pour sauce into blender. Season to taste and puree to smooth consistency.
4. Serve hot on the plate with the Salmon Mousse, if desired. Any remaining sauce can be refrigerated or frozen.

YIELD: 2 CUPS

Grilled Tomato with Rosemary

DAY 3

1 large ripe tomato
1 teaspoon chopped fresh rosemary, or ¼ teaspoon dried
1 clove garlic, crushed
Freshly ground pepper to taste

1. Preheat the broiler.
2. Rinse and dry the tomato. Do not core or peel. Split tomato in half crosswise and arrange halves on a baking dish.
3. Chop the rosemary coarsely and combine with

251

crushed garlic to form paste. Sprinkle on the cut surface of the tomato. Dust with pepper.

    4. Broil the tomato 4 to 5 inches away from the flame for about 3 minutes or until garlic is browned. Then place in 400° F. oven for 6 to 8 minutes.

    5. Serve hot.

2 SERVINGS (1 SERVING = ½ TOMATO)

Croque-Monsieur
(Melted Cheese Sandwich)

DAY 4

2 *slices French bread (3½″ x 2¼″ x ½″ thin)*
4 *ounces skim-milk cheese (i.e., Jarlsberg or Valembert)*

    1. Toast bread lightly on both sides under broiler.

    2. Place thin slices of cheese on toasted bread. Broil until cheese melts. Serve hot.

2 SERVINGS (1 SERVING = 1 SLICE)

Broccoli Vinaigrette

DAY 4

1 *cup broccoli flowerettes*
2 *tablespoons freshly squeezed lemon juice*
½ *teaspoon Dijon mustard*
½ *clove garlic, smashed*
Salt and freshly ground pepper to taste
Optional: pinch of dried herb such as basil

    1. Steam broccoli (page 238) until tender, but still crisp, about 5 to 8 minutes. Drain. Place in a bowl with cold

water and let stand until thoroughly cool. Refrigerate for 1 to 2 hours or overnight.

2. To prepare the vinaigrette, mix together lemon juice, mustard, garlic, salt and pepper and, if desired, the dried herb.

3. Spoon mixture over the cold broccoli and serve, or let broccoli marinate in it for at least 1 hour.

2 SERVINGS (1 SERVING = ½ CUP)

Steamed Fillet of Sole with Fennel

DAYS 4 AND 5

1 pound fillet of sole
1 tablespoon chopped shallots
1 teaspoon (½ clove) minced garlic
¼–½ teaspoon crumbled fennel seeds, or 1 tablespoon
    chopped fresh dill
Salt and freshly ground pepper to taste
1 tablespoon vermouth, or 2 tablespoons dry white wine

1. Wash and dry fish and place it on a heatproof plate just large enough to hold it. Sprinkle the shallots, seasonings and wine over the fish.

2. Use a wok with a cover or improvise a steamer as follows: Set a baking or roasting pan on the burner and stand a metal trivet in the middle to hold the plate. Set the plate on the trivet and pour boiling water into the pan, but not enough to reach the plate. Cover the top of the pan (and the fish on the plate) with aluminum foil and crimp the edges to seal it tightly. Put the burner on low heat to keep the water simmering.

3. Cook until done—about 10 minutes—and serve immediately with the fish juices. Refrigerate remaining fish.

5 SERVINGS: 3 DINNER (4 OUNCES EACH) AND 2 LUNCH (2 OUNCES EACH)

Poached Pears in Wine
DAYS 4 AND 7

1 *cup water*
½ *cup white wine*
1 *cinnamon stick*
1 *slice lemon*
Pinch of ground nutmeg
2 *ripe pears, peeled, halved, cored*

1. In a small saucepan bring the water, wine, cinnamon stick, lemon and nutmeg to boil over moderate heat.
2. Add pears; cover and simmer 15 to 20 minutes until pears are just tender. Remove cinnamon stick and reserve.
3. Chill pears in juice several hours before serving. Garnish with cinnamon stick.

2 SERVINGS (1 SERVING = 1 PEAR)

Cold Asparagus with Roquefort
DAY 5

1 *cup fresh asparagus*
¼ *tablespoon Roquefort cheese*
2 *tablespoons lemon juice*
Freshly ground pepper to taste
Lettuce or other greens (unlimited quantity)

1. Trim off the tough white end of asparagus stalks with a paring knife. Steam briefly (see page 238) until tender, about 5 minutes, then cool.
2. Disperse cheese in lemon juice (a little water may be used to extend mixture) and add pepper to taste.
3. Arrange asparagus on bed of escarole, chicory, wa-

254

tercress or romaine lettuce. Dress with Roquefort-lemon juice mixture.

2 SERVINGS (1 SERVING = ½ CUP)

Veau à la Provençale
(Veal Cutlets)

DAY 5

½ cup chicken or veal stock
2 4-ounce veal cutlets (⅓"–½" thick), or 8 ounces veal
    cubes
1 clove garlic, minced
1 cup peeled, seeded and chopped tomatoes
Garnish: chopped parsley

1. Heat 2 tablespoons chicken or veal stock in a seasoned nonstick pan, brown cutlets or cubes on both sides. Add garlic, tomatoes and chicken or veal stock. Cover and simmer for 15 to 20 minutes.

2. Sprinkle with parsley and serve. Liquid may be further reduced if necessary.

2 SERVINGS (1 SERVING = 1 CUTLET OR 4 OUNCES VEAL CUBES)

Braised Leeks

DAY 5

4 leeks, white portion only, washed well
1½–2 cups canned or homemade chicken stock
Salt and freshly ground pepper
1 tablespoon finely chopped fresh parsley

1. Cut the stalks of the leeks in half lengthwise, then in half crosswise.

2. In a skillet, heat the chicken stock until it boils. Add the leeks and salt and freshly ground pepper. Cover and simmer until the leeks are tender, about 10 to 15 minutes.

3. Serve half the leeks hot or cold with a sprinkling of chopped fresh parsley.

4. For cold braised leek salad, sprinkle on 1 tablespoon lemon juice (freshly squeezed) and then the parsley. Chill for several hours. Serve.

4 SERVINGS (1 SERVING = ½ CUP)

Onion Soup

DAY 6

1 *extra-large Bermuda onion, thinly sliced*
4 cups homemade or canned chicken broth
Freshly ground pepper
¼ cup dry sherry
4 ounces sliced skim-milk mozzarella cheese

1. Sauté onion carefully in covered nonstick pan over low to medium heat until tender but not brown, adding a few tablespoons of water or chicken broth when necessary.

2. Heat chicken broth in separate saucepan. Add onion and pepper and simmer for ½ hour.

3. Before serving, add ¼ cup dry sherry. Heat thoroughly for 5 minutes.

4. Place in crocks topped with 1 ounce thinly sliced skim-milk mozzarella cheese. Place under hot broiler for 5 to 7 minutes, until cheese melts. Serve immediately.

4 SERVINGS (1 SERVING = 1 CUP)

Sliced Tomatoes with Cucumber Sauce

DAY 6

1 cup tomato slices

CUCUMBER SAUCE
Juice of ½ lemon
2 tablespoons cold water
2 medium Kirby cucumbers, peeled, seeded and cut into
   pieces
½ teaspoon Dijon mustard
¼ teaspoon chopped fresh basil, or ⅛ teaspoon dried (or
   same amounts of other fresh or dried herbs such as dill)
1 tablespoon fresh parsley
1 clove garlic, smashed
Salt and freshly ground pepper to taste
Garnish: watercress and 1 tablespoon capers (optional)

1. Arrange tomato slices on an oval plate, letting them slightly overlap each other. Chill in refrigerator.

2. Prepare Cucumber Sauce by adding lemon juice and water to blender, then cucumber pieces, mustard, basil and parsley. Puree until cucumber turns into thick sauce. Add garlic and season with salt and pepper.

3. Refrigerate 30 minutes. Spoon over tomato slices and garnish with watercress and capers.

2 SERVINGS (1 SERVING = ½ CUP TOMATO SLICES)

Moules à la Marinière
(Fresh Mussels in Wine)

DAY 6

40 *small to medium mussels*
1 *cup dry white vermouth, or 2 cups dry white wine*
½ *cup minced shallots or green onions or finely minced*
  onions
8 *parsley sprigs*
½ *bay leaf*
½ *teaspoon dried thyme*
⅛ *teaspoon freshly ground black pepper*
½ *cup coarsely chopped parsley*

1. Scrub the mussels well with a stiff brush and scrape the tuft of hairs or beard with a small knife. Wash them in cold water, soaking them for an hour or two. Discard any mussels that are not firmly closed or feel lighter in weight (or even heavier) than the rest.

2. Bring the vermouth or wine to a boil in large enameled pot with the shallots or onion, parsley sprigs, bay leaf, thyme and pepper. Boil for 2 to 3 minutes to evaporate the wine's alcohol content and reduce it slightly.

3. Add the mussels to the pot, cover tightly with its lid and boil quickly over high heat. Hold onto the cover and the handles or sides of the pot with both hands and toss the mussels frequently with an up-and-down, jerky motion. This will allow all the mussels to cook evenly. The mussel shells should open in about 5 minutes and will be done. Discard any that do not open.

4. Remove the mussels with a slotted spoon into soup plates and let the cooking liquid settle a minute or so. Then ladle liquid over mussels and sprinkle with chopped parsley. Serve immediately.

2 SERVINGS (1 SERVING = 20 MUSSELS)

Fruit et Fromage
(Fruit and Cheese Plate)

DAY 7

2 ounces skim-milk cheese (i.e., Valembert or French
    Royal Morbier) or 2 ounces skim-milk ricotta
1 fresh pear
Bed of Boston or Bibb lettuce

Thinly slice the cheese and the pear and arrange on lettuce bed. Cheese can be placed (or spread) on top of the fruit and eaten that way.

1 SERVING

Bouillabaisse
(Fish Stew)

DAY 7

½ pound raw shrimp
½ teaspoon olive oil
2 cloves garlic, finely chopped
1 cup chopped onion
1 teaspoon chicken or vegetable bouillon
4 cups peeled fresh or canned tomatoes
½ cup dry white vermouth
½ teaspoon hot pepper flakes
1 teaspoon dried thyme
2 teaspoons dried basil
1 teaspoon crumbled saffron
2 whole cloves
Salt and freshly ground pepper to taste
¾ pound white-fleshed fish (such as cod or striped bass),
    cut into large pieces
20 clams
1 tablespoon Pernod or Ricard (vodka can be substituted)

259

1. Clean and shell the shrimp and set aside.
2. Season a nonstick pan with oil, heat, and then cook garlic over medium heat for 30 seconds. Carefully slide in onion and then add chicken or vegetable bouillon.
3. Add tomatoes and vermouth and then the pepper flakes, thyme, basil, saffron, cloves and salt and pepper to taste.
4. Bring to a boil, then pour into food processor or blender and puree.
5. Return to skillet, cover and cook 15 minutes. Add shrimp, fish and clams and simmer, partly covered, for 20 minutes longer.
6. Add Pernod or Ricard and cook 10 minutes more.
7. Serve piping hot in heated soup plates.

6 SERVINGS (1 SERVING = 4 OUNCES TOTAL OF SHRIMP AND FISH INCLUDING 3 CLAMS)

Gratin aux Zucchini
(Zucchini with Cheese)

DAY 7

1 *cup thinly sliced tender zucchini, peeled*
2 *ounces skim-milk mozzarella cheese, cubed*
1 *tablespoon grated Parmesan cheese*
1 *sprig fresh parsley, chopped*
2 *tablespoons bread crumbs*

1. Preheat oven to 350° F.
2. Put a third of the zucchini into a nonstick baking dish, then a third each of the mozzarella cubes, Parmesan cheese, and parsley. Make more layers in this manner, using the remaining ingredients. Cover with bread crumbs.
3. Bake, uncovered, until golden brown, about 30 minutes. Serve hot.

2 SERVINGS (1 SERVING = ½ CUP ZUCCHINI)

260

Italian Recipes

Antipasto Salad

DAY 1

*Bed of mixed greens (unlimited quantity): chicory,
    escarole, arugula*
Italian Dressing (page 262)
*2 ounces Cooked Turkey Breast (see page 237), cubed or
    sliced*
2 ounces skim-milk mozzarella cheese, sliced
1 cup fresh tomato wedges

1. Wash and dry greens and place in a large mixing bowl.

2. Pour on a few tablespoons of the dressing and toss the greens until coated.

3. Arrange on a plate with the other ingredients and spoon on a few more tablespoons of the dressing.

2 SERVINGS (1 SERVING = 2 OUNCES TOTAL OF TURKEY AND MOZZARELLA, ½ CUP TOMATO WEDGES)

Italian Dressing

3 tablespoons wine vinegar or fresh lemon juice
½ small onion, peeled
1 clove garlic, peeled
1 teaspoon dried oregano or basil leaves
½ teaspoon salt
⅛ teaspoon pepper
½ cup water

1. Put first six ingredients into electric blender; cover and puree at high speed until smooth.
2. Add water and blend again at low speed.
3. Keep dressing in refrigerator and shake before using.

NOTE: If you don't care for a strong garlic flavor, don't blend the garlic with the other ingredients. Rather, smash the clove of garlic and add it to the dressing after it is blended.

YIELD: ⅔ CUP

Shrimp Marinara

DAY 1

½ pound shrimp
2 cups (½ recipe) Light Tomato Sauce
1 cup hot cooked linguini

LIGHT TOMATO SAUCE

1 35-ounce can Italian plum tomatoes, or 4 pounds fresh
   plum tomatoes, halved
½ teaspoon dried basil, or 2 leaves of fresh
½ teaspoon dried oregano

262

2–3 cloves garlic, mashed
½ cup dry red or white wine
Freshly ground black pepper to taste
(Yields: approximately 4 cups)

1. Shell, devein and wash shrimp.
2. To prepare sauce, place the tomatoes, basil, oregano, garlic and wine in a deep saucepan with a cover and simmer slowly (20 minutes for the canned tomatoes and 1 hour for the fresh). Remove the pan from the heat and remove garlic with a fork or spoon.
3. Chop coarsely in electric blender or pass through food mill. Season with freshly ground pepper. (The remainder can be frozen until ready to use.)
4. Bring sauce to a boil, add shrimp and reduce heat at once. Simmer, covered, 3 to 5 minutes.
5. Spoon sauce over linguini and place the shrimp on top. Serve hot.

2 SERVINGS (1 SERVING = 4 OUNCES SHRIMP AND ½ CUP LINGUINI)

Cappuccino

¼ cup skim milk, warmed
2 cups freshly brewed, decaffeinated espresso
Cinnamon

1. Whip the skim milk with a wire whisk until frothy, or blend in an electric blender.
2. Fill two drinking cups three-quarters of the way with hot coffee. Top each cup with the whipped skim milk.
3. Sprinkle with cinnamon. Serve hot.

2 SERVINGS

263

Pizza Southampton

DAY 2

2 *slices extra-large tomato, or 2–3 tablespoons Light*
  Tomato Sauce (page 262)
2 *ounces skim-milk mozzarella cheese, sliced*
1 *whole-wheat pita bread, split in round halves*
Dash oregano

1. Preheat oven to 500° F.
2. Place tomato slice or tomato sauce and then mozzarella cheese on each half of the open pita bread. Season with oregano.
3. Place on cookie sheet and heat in oven until the pita bread is crispy and the cheese is melted and slightly bubbly —about 8 minutes. Serve hot.

1 SERVING

Garlic Broiled Turkey or Veal

DAY 2

1–2 *cloves garlic*
½ *teaspoon kosher (coarse) salt*
8 *ounces turkey breast cutlets, sliced, or 8 ounces veal*
  cubes
2 *tablespoons chicken stock (optional, for turkey)*

1. Preheat broiler to medium/high.
2. Peel and chop garlic. Sprinkle salt over garlic pieces and crush salt into garlic with the side of knife, scraping and crushing until all the salt is absorbed into garlic.
3. Line baking pan with foil and arrange turkey or veal. Sprinkle fresh garlic salt over pieces, grinding into and across the grain of meat.

4. Place under broiler for 5 to 8 minutes, until meat turns color. Turn and cook unseasoned side. For last 2 to 3 minutes of cooking time, turn meat again, spoon over chicken stock (if necessary) and turn broiler to high. This promotes browning, but be sure not to burn. Serve hot.

2 SERVINGS (1 SERVING = 4 OUNCES TURKEY BREAST OR VEAL CUBES)

Broccoli or Green Bean Salad

DAYS 2 AND 6

1 cup fresh broccoli flowerettes
1–2 tablespoons freshly squeezed lemon juice
1 clove garlic, quartered
Salt and freshly ground pepper to taste

1. Steam broccoli (see page 238) until tender (8 to 10 minutes).

2. Immediately remove the broccoli from the steamer and place in a bowl of ice-cold water. Let stand 5 to 10 minutes until quite cold. (This helps to retain the dark-green color and crisp texture.) Drain.

3. Combine lemon juice and garlic. Wait 10 minutes. Discard garlic.

4. Sprinkle broccoli with salt, freshly ground pepper, and garlic-flavored lemon juice. Chill 1 hour before serving.

NOTE: For Green Bean Salad, steam 1 cup of whole fresh beans for approximately 10 to 15 minutes or until tender. Follow same instructions as for broccoli.

2 SERVINGS (1 SERVING = ½ CUP BROCCOLI FLOW-ERETTES OR STRING BEANS)

Tonno
(Tuna Salad)

DAY 3

1 cup (7 ounces) canned tuna (packed in water, drained)
Freshly ground pepper to taste
2 tablespoons wine vinegar
1 cup tomato wedges
2 thin slices Spanish onion
2 tablespoons chopped celery
Cucumber, thinly sliced (unlimited)
Bed of romaine or leaf lettuce (unlimited)
Garnish: 4 thin slices green or red sweet pepper

1. Place tuna in salad bowl, add pepper and vinegar, toss, add vegetables and toss again.
2. Serve on a bed of romaine or leaf lettuce. Garnish with green or red pepper.

2 SERVINGS (1 SERVING = ½ CUP TUNA, ½ CUP TOMATO WEDGES)

Grilled Bluefish

DAY 3

1 pound bluefish fillets
¼ cup red wine
1 clove garlic, crushed
Juice of ½ fresh lemon
Freshly ground pepper to taste
Garnish: chopped fresh parsley and ½ fresh lemon, peeled and thinly sliced

1. Preheat oven to 350° F.
2. Cut fish fillets into squares and marinate in red wine, garlic and lemon juice for 20 minutes.

266

3. Cut four pieces of heavy-duty aluminum foil to approximately 12" x 12" each. Place two smaller sheets of grease-proof paper in the center of each.

4. Divide fish into four portions and place each in the center of a sheet. Season with black pepper and garnish with chopped parsley and lemon slices. Pull together edges of paper and then crimp foil to make a loose parcel. Fold short ends together tight.

5. Place in oven for 10 to 15 minutes, or cook for 10 minutes on hot charcoal grill.

NOTE: Mackerel or shad fillets may be substituted for bluefish.

4 SERVINGS (1 SERVING = 4 OUNCES)

Sliced Tomato Salad with Basil and Oregano

DAY 3

1 cup sliced fresh tomatoes
1 teaspoon chopped fresh basil, or ¼ teaspoon dried
¼ teaspoon dried oregano
2 tablespoons freshly squeezed lemon juice
1 clove garlic, smashed
Salt and freshly ground pepper to taste
Garnish: 1 teaspoon chopped parsley

1. Arrange the tomato slices on a platter.

2. Blend together the basil, oregano, lemon juice and garlic. Remove garlic with a fork or spoon.

3. Pour mixture over the tomatoes. Season with salt and pepper.

4. Garnish with chopped parsley and serve.

2 SERVINGS (1 SERVING = ½ CUP SLICED TOMATOES)

267

Crostini
(Toasted Cheese Sandwich)
DAY 4

1 *medium slice of whole-wheat Italian bread*
1 *ounce turkey, sliced*
1 *ounce skim-milk mozzarella cheese, sliced*
1 *slice of tomato (optional)*

1. Toast the bread on both sides under the broiler.
2. Place a slice of turkey on the toasted bread and top with sliced mozzarella. If a tomato slice is desired, place it on the toasted bread first.
3. Grill under the broiler several inches from the flame until cheese melts. Serve hot.

1 SERVING

Artichoke Salad
DAY 4

2 *fresh medium artichokes*
½ *lemon*
2 *tablespoons lemon juice*
2 *tablespoons flour*
Italian Dressing (page 262), or 1 tablespoon lemon juice
Bed of salad greens (unlimited)

1. Wash the artichokes thoroughly in cold water, cut off the stem, flush with the base, with a stainless steel knife. Remove the tough outer leaves with your hands and trim off about 1 inch of the top. Rub a lemon half on cut edges to prevent discoloration. With a pair of scissors snip off the tip of each leaf and rub cut edges with lemon. To remove the hairy fibers and the choke, use a knife or a sharp-edged metal spoon and cut

around the inside and scoop it out. Squeeze lemon juice in empty cavity.

2. Bring about 2 quarts of water plus the lemon juice and flour to a boil in an enamel, stainless steel or glass pan. Add the artichokes and return water to boil. Cook until tender, approximately 20 to 40 minutes. Remove the artichokes from the pan and place on plates.

3. Spoon a few tablespoons of dressing over each artichoke or sprinkle with fresh lemon juice. Serve hot or chilled on a bed of greens.

2 SERVINGS (1 SERVING = 1 ARTICHOKE)

Grilled Chicken

DAY 4

1 *whole (8-ounce) chicken breast, or 8 ounces Cornish hen*
1 *clove garlic, split*
1 *teaspoon kosher (coarse) salt*
Freshly ground pepper
Garnish: 2 tablespoons chopped Italian parsley, lemon wedges

1. Split the chicken breast or Cornish hen in half (but do not cut completely through). Open the breast or hen and flatten it out with your hands. Rub the skin with the garlic clove.

2. Heat broiler. Place the chicken or Cornish hen on a rack over a broiling pan. Season with the salt and pepper. (The chicken can also be charcoal broiled.) Broil for 8 to 10 minutes, turn it over and cook for approximately 8 to 10 minutes more. Test with a fork for doneness and, if it's not completely cooked through, return it again to the broiler.

3. Remove the skin before serving, and garnish with chopped parsley and lemon wedges.

2 SERVINGS (1 SERVING = 4 OUNCES CHICKEN)

Veal Burger

DAY 5

4 ounces ground veal
2 pinches of oregano
Freshly ground black pepper to taste
2 slices whole-wheat Italian bread
2 tablespoons Light Tomato Sauce (page 262) (optional)

1. Mix veal, oregano and pepper together. Divide in half and shape into patties.
2. Broil burgers on medium 6 to 8 minutes each side until done.
3. Serve on slice of whole-wheat Italian bread. (Optional: Spoon a tablespoon of Light Tomato Sauce on top of each burger.)

2 SERVINGS (1 SERVING = 2 OUNCES VEAL; 1 SLICE BREAD)

Spigola Bollito (Poached Bass)

DAYS 5 AND 6

2½ cups water
½ cup white wine
1 tablespoon vinegar
Juice of ½ lemon, retain peel
½ carrot, finely chopped
½ medium onion, finely chopped
¼ knob celeriac, or 1 rib of celery, finely chopped
1 bay leaf
4 peppercorns
Pinch of salt
1¼–1½ pounds striped bass
8 boiled new potatoes
Garnish: lemon wedges

1. Prepare court-bouillon in a fish poacher, using water, wine, vinegar, lemon juice, vegetables, bay leaf, peppercorns and salt. If you don't have a fish poacher, use a large saucepan with a steaming rack and a piece of cheesecloth laid across the steamer, allowing cloth to hang over edges of the pan.

2. Cover pan and boil bouillon for 30 minutes over medium heat, adding more water if it evaporates and skimming carefully. Cool at room temperature.

3. Wash and dry fish, rub with inside of squeezed lemon half.

4. Place fish on rack, bring liquid to boil and steam for 5 to 8 minutes until fish flakes easily with fork.

5. Remove from pan carefully and serve on oval platter with boiled new potatoes and lemon wedges. Spoon 2 to 3 tablespoons fish stock over dish.

6. Chill leftover fish to be eaten cold (with lemon wedges) for lunch the following day.

SERVINGS: 4 DINNERS (4 OUNCES EACH) AND 2 LUNCHES (2 OUNCES EACH)

Roasted Red Pepper Salad

DAY 5

1 *medium sweet red pepper*
1 *tablespoon fresh lemon juice*
1 *clove garlic, mashed*
2 *teaspoons finely chopped fresh basil, oregano or parsley*
Salt and freshly ground pepper to taste

1. Broil whole pepper for 4 to 10 minutes about 2 inches from the heat, spearing pepper with a fork. Turn the pepper as its skin blisters to broil it evenly. Remove from heat.

2. Immediately peel away the skin, holding pepper over a plate with tongs to catch any juices. Do not let the pepper cool or it becomes too difficult to peel the skin—but be careful not to burn your fingers. Remove the stem and the cluster of seeds with a spoon. Save the pepper juices remaining on the plate.

3. Mix together the lemon juice, garlic, reserved pepper juice and basil, oregano or parsley or shake well in a covered jar. Remove the garlic.

4. Lay the pepper, peeled side up, on a plate and pour the dressing over it. Season with salt and pepper.

5. Serve the salad immediately, or for improved flavor let it marinate for several hours at room temperature.

2 SERVINGS (1 SERVING = ½ CUP PEPPER)

Zuppa di Vongole or di Cozze (Clam or Mussel Soup)

DAY 6

40 *small clams or mussels*
1 *small leek, white part only (thoroughly washed and chopped)*
1 *cup finely chopped onion*
1 *cup dry white wine*
1 *8-ounce can peeled Italian plum tomatoes, crushed*
2–3 *cloves garlic, crushed*
½ *teaspoon dried oregano*
½ *cup chopped parsley*

1. Scrub clams or mussels thoroughly in cold running water. Then soak for 1 hour in fresh cold salted water until clams or mussels are completely sand-free.

2. Sauté leek and onion in a nonstick saucepan until just brown.

3. Drain the clams or mussels, add to pan, cover and cook for 5 minutes over brisk heat.

272

4. Add wine, tomatoes, garlic, oregano and parsley. Cook again for 5 minutes or until clams or mussels are fully open; discard any that are closed. Serve in soup bowls with liquid.

2 SERVINGS (1 SERVING = 20 CLAMS OR MUSSELS)

DAY 6

1 *small orange, sectioned*
12 *green grapes*
2 *dried or fresh figs, cut up*
½ *banana, sliced*
Garnish: 4 mint leaves

1. Mix fruit. Spoon into wineglasses or goblets.
2. Serve chilled, garnished with a mint leaf.

4 SERVINGS (1 SERVING = ½ CUP APPROXIMATELY)

Sliced Tomatoes and Mozzarella Cheese with Basil

DAY 7

1 *cup sliced fresh tomatoes*
4 *ounces skim-milk mozzarella cheese, sliced*
1 *teaspoon chopped fresh basil, or ¼ teaspoon dried basil*
Salt and freshly ground pepper to taste

1. Arrange the tomato slices and sliced mozzarella by alternating 1 slice of tomato with 1 slice of mozzarella until all slices are used.
2. Season with basil and salt and pepper to taste.
3. Serve at room temperature.

2 SERVINGS (1 SERVING = ½ CUP SLICED TOMATOES, 2 OUNCES MOZZARELLA)

273

Codfish Steaks in Tomato Sauce

DAY 7

4–5 *fresh plum tomatoes, peeled and chopped, or 1 cup*
chopped canned plum tomatoes
2 sprigs parsley, chopped
¼ cup dry white wine
½ pound codfish steaks (1 large or 2 medium)
Salt and freshly ground pepper to taste

1. Cook the tomatoes, chopped parsley and wine over medium heat until it is a thick sauce—about 20 minutes.
2. Add fish steaks, cover and cook for 5 to 10 minutes, depending on size. Season with salt and pepper to taste.
3. Remove fish carefully when serving.

2 SERVINGS (1 SERVING = 4 OUNCES FISH)

Garlic-Flavored Spinach

DAY 7

½ pound fresh spinach (young and tender)
¼ cup chicken bouillon
1 clove garlic, smashed
Lemon juice
Freshly ground pepper to taste

1. Remove the stems from the spinach leaves and discard any imperfect leaves. Wash the spinach quickly in a bowl with several changes of cold water until it is completely sand-free.
2. Heat the bouillon and garlic for 2 to 3 minutes in a nonstick pan. Add spinach. Cover at once and cook over high

heat until steam appears. Reduce the heat and simmer until tender, about 5 to 6 minutes.

3. Discard garlic, using a fork or spoon, and season with lemon juice and pepper to taste. Serve immediately.

2 SERVINGS (1 SERVING = ½ CUP)

Japanese Recipes

Three-Flavor Vinegar Crab or Shrimp Salad

DAYS 1 AND 3

1 *cucumber, thinly sliced or more, if desired*
3 *teaspoons salt dissolved in 1½ cups water*
1 *cup chilled canned or fresh cooked crabmeat*
*Garnish: sprig of watercress and thin tomato slice or
carrot curl*

FLAVORED VINEGAR DRESSING
2 *tablespoons rice vinegar*
2 *tablespoons soy sauce (preferably light—otherwise use
1¾ tablespoons dark and ¼ tablespoon water)*
2 *teaspoons fresh ginger juice (see page 262)*

1. Soak cucumber in salted water for 15 to 20 minutes. Pour off water and squeeze cucumber to drain any remaining liquid. Cucumber slices should be limp and slightly salty.

2. To make dressing, mix rice vinegar and soy sauce in pan over medium heat. Bring just to boil. Remove from heat and cool to room temperature. Squeeze ginger root in garlic press to make ginger juice. Add fresh ginger juice and mix well.

3. Arrange crabmeat in center of plate, surrounded by slices of prepared cucumber; and spoon vinegar dressing over plate. Garnish with watercress sprig and tomato or carrot for color. Serve chilled.

NOTE: For Three-Flavor Vinegar Shrimp Salad substitute 10 cooked small or 5 medium shrimp (either fresh or frozen) for the crabmeat.

2 SERVINGS (1 SERVING = ½ CUP CRABMEAT)

Chicken Teriyaki

DAY 1

8 ounces chicken breasts, skinned and boned
½ cup Teriyaki Sauce
⅓ cup sectioned red peppers
⅓ cup sliced zucchini
⅓ cup halved mushrooms
Dash of freshly ground pepper
Garnish: ginger root, cut into slivers

TERIYAKI SAUCE
7 tablespoons sake
7 tablespoons light or dark soy sauce
7 tablespoons dry white wine
½ teaspoon finely chopped ginger root
(Yields 1⅓ cups)

1. Cut chicken into ½" to 1" cubes.
2. To prepare sauce, combine ingredients and mix well. (Sauce can be made ahead and kept, covered, in refrigerator for a few days. Unused portion can also be stored.)
3. Marinate chicken in Teriyaki Sauce for 30 minutes, turning pieces to absorb flavor.
4. Line baking pan with foil and place under broiler to preheat. Turn meat in marinade one last time before putting into pan to cook.
5. Marinate prepared vegetables in sauce while chicken is cooking.
6. Place chicken in baking pan and under broiler. Turn the chicken every 2 to 3 minutes, basting with a little of the sauce until done, approximately 8 minutes. The outside will be dark brown, but not burnt, while inside flesh is white and succulent.
7. Remove chicken from pan, and fill the pan with the marinated vegetables. Broil vegetable pieces for 3 to 4 minutes until hot but still crisp.

8. Meanwhile, pour rest of marinade into medium-hot nonstick frying pan and bring liquid to boil while stirring. After a minute or so the liquid will thicken slightly and take on a luster. Place chicken in frying pan and continue cooking for another minute over a high heat. Stir and turn meat so that it is well coated with the reduced sauce.

9. Add dash of black pepper and serve with hot vegetables and small side dish of ginger root slivers.

2 SERVINGS (1 SERVING = 4 OUNCES CHICKEN, ½ CUP VEGETABLES)

White Rice

This recipe produces a moist rice, the kind that is typically served with an Oriental meal. It is used in the Japanese and Chinese menus of this book and in some of the other ethnic recipes.

½ cup long-grain rice
1½ cups water or stock (fish, vegetable, veal, beef or chicken to coincide with main course)

1. Combine rice and water or stock in a small saucepan.

2. Bring mixture to a boil, uncovered, and immediately reduce heat to low simmer. Shake pot and cover tightly.

3. Cook until all the liquid is absorbed—about 10 to 15 minutes. Remove from heat and let stand 5 minutes.

4. Serve immediately.

3 SERVINGS (1 SERVING = ½ CUP)

Simmered String Beans or Carrots
DAYS 1 AND 7

1 cup string beans, halved, or 1 cup carrots, peeled and
   cut into 2" julienne strips
2 tablespoons sake
2 tablespoons soy sauce
½ teaspoon toasted sesame seeds (page 162)
Garnish: 2 red pepper rings and sprig of parsley or
   watercress

1. Steam string beans or carrots over water (see page 238) for 5 minutes. Test with sharp knife—outside should be softened while center is still firm. Empty water from pan and let vegetable drain in the steamer while making sauce.

2. Meanwhile, pour sake in pan and boil off the alcohol. Stir in soy sauce and continue cooking until liquid has been reduced by half. Gently slide string beans or carrots into this sauce and heat for 30 seconds. Sprinkle with toasted sesame seeds.

3. Serve hot. Garnish with red pepper rings and sprig of parsley or watercress.

2 SERVINGS (1 SERVING = ½ CUP VEGETABLES)

Chicken and Asparagus (or Broccoli) Salad with Mustard Dressing

DAY 2

4 ounces Cooked (boiled or poached) Chicken Breast (see
    page 237), boned, skinned and cut into pieces
1 cup steamed asparagus spears (see page 238), cut into
    ½" lengths, or 1 cup steamed fresh broccoli spears, cut
    into pieces
Garnish: watercress sprigs and 2 tomato wedges

MUSTARD DRESSING

½ teaspoon powdered mustard (mixed with ½ teaspoon
    water)
1 tablespoon light soy sauce
1–2 tablespoons rice vinegar
¼ teaspoon grated fresh ginger

1. Place the cooked chicken and asparagus (or broccoli) in a bowl.

2. Prepare Mustard Dressing by mixing the ingredients together well.

3. Add the dressing to the chicken and vegetable. Toss lightly to coat all the ingredients.

4. Serve warm or cold. Garnish each plate with sprigs of watercress and a tomato wedge.

2 SERVINGS (1 SERVING = 2 OUNCES CHICKEN, ½ CUP VEGETABLES)

Sake Simmered Fish

DAY 2

4 *tablespoons dry white wine*
1 *tablespoon sake*
¾ *cup dashi (chicken broth)*
3 *tablespoons soy sauce*
1 *pound halibut or turbot, cut into steaks and boned*
Garnish: sprig parsley or watercress, and radish or thin
    tomato slice

1. Mix wine and sake in medium-size skillet and boil over high heat to eliminate alcohol. Stir in dashi and soy sauce and bring to boil.

2. Carefully lay fish in stock and cover immediately. Cook for approximately 10 minutes in boiling liquid. This quick-cook method keeps fish delicate and fragrant.

3. Carefully lift fish pieces onto plate and spoon liquid on top. Garnish with parsley or watercress, and radish or thin tomato slice.

NOTE: This dish is excellent hot, but can also be served chilled, in which case the broth will jell. Refrigerated it keeps for up to 2 days, and may be reheated in seasoned broth and, if necessary, a little water.

4 SERVINGS (1 SERVING = 4 OUNCES)

Green Beans, Spinach or Cucumbers and Radishes with Sesame Dressing
DAYS 2, 5 AND 6

1 cup steamed green beans (see page 238), or ½ pound
    parboiled fresh spinach, cut into 1½" lengths, or sliced
    cucumbers and radishes (unlimited)
Garnish: thin tomato slice or carrot curl

SESAME DRESSING
½ teaspoon toasted sesame seeds (see page 162)
1 tablespoon light or dark soy sauce
1½ tablespoons dashi (chicken bouillon)

1. Prepare dressing by mixing sesame seeds with soy
sauce and dashi.
2. Pour dressing over hot (cooked) green beans or
spinach (arranged on a plate) or raw cucumbers and radishes.
Garnish with tomato or carrot for color.

2 SERVINGS (1 SERVING = ½ CUP)

Chicken Yakitori with Vegetables
DAY 3

8 ounces chicken breasts, skinned, boned and cut into 1"
    pieces
4 scallions, cut into 2" lengths
¼ cup sectioned sweet red pepper
¼ cup sliced zucchini
¼ cup halved mushrooms and 4 whole mushrooms
4 bamboo skewers

YAKITORI SAUCE

¼ cup light or dark soy sauce
¼ cup dry white wine
¼ teaspoon finely grated ginger root
1 tablespoon lemon juice

1. Line a baking pan with foil and preheat under broiler.

2. Combine soy sauce, wine, ginger root, and lemon juice and marinate chicken, scallions and other vegetables except whole mushrooms for 20 to 30 minutes. Turn them twice so that the flavor is completely absorbed.

3. Alternate chicken with scallions on each bamboo skewer, turn skewer in sauce one last time. Separate caps from stems of whole mushrooms and place a mushroom cap at the end of each skewer.

4. Place the mushroom stems and vegetables in preheated baking pan and then place skewers on top. Spoon some sauce over before returning to broiler.

5. Turn skewers every 2 to 3 minutes, basting chicken with a little of the sauce. Chicken will be cooked in 6 to 8 minutes. The outside will be dark brown (but not burnt) while inside flesh is white and succulent.

6. Remove skewers from heat and arrange on plate while vegetables cook an extra minute or two. Serve hot.

2 SERVINGS (1 SERVING — 4 OUNCES CHICKEN AND ½ CUP VEGETABLES)

Chicken and Beansprout or Chicken and Cucumber Salad with Sesame Dressing

DAYS 4 AND 7

¾ cup beansprouts, blanched (see instructions below), or
  ¾ cup peeled, thinly sliced cucumbers, or more, if
  desired
4 ounces Cooked Chicken Breast (page 237), shredded
1 teaspoon finely sliced scallions
¼ cup shredded green pepper
Bed of lettuce (unlimited)

SESAME DRESSING
½ teaspoon sesame seeds, toasted (page 162)
2 tablespoons light or dark soy sauce
3 tablespoons dashi (chicken bouillon)

1. Blanch the beansprouts: Place them in a bowl and pour over boiling water. Drain the hot water immediately and cover the beansprouts with cool water. This preserves their crispness. The sprouts are drained again and dried with paper towels before using. To keep the cucumbers crisp, first soak the slices in salted water (3 teaspoons of salt dissolved in 1½ cups water). Pour off the water and squeeze the cucumbers to drain any liquid. The cucumbers should be limp and slightly salty.

2. Mix together the ingredients for Sesame Dressing.

3. Add chicken, blanched beansprouts, scallions and green pepper to bowl. Pour dressing and toss to coat ingredients evenly. Serve on bed of lettuce.

2 SERVINGS (1 SERVING = 2 OUNCES CHICKEN AND ½ CUP VEGETABLES)

Scallops Yakitori with Vegetables

DAY 4

1 *recipe Yakitori Sauce (page 283)*
½ pound sea scallops
4 scallions, cut into 2" lengths
⅓ cup sectioned red pepper
⅓ cup sliced zucchini
⅓ cup halved mushrooms
4 bamboo skewers

1. Line a baking pan with foil and preheat under broiler.

2. Combine ingredients for sauce and marinate scallops, scallions and other vegetables for 20–30 minutes. Turn them twice so that the flavor is completely absorbed.

3. Alternate scallops with scallions on bamboo skewer, turn in sauce one last time.

4. Place vegetables in preheated baking pan and then place skewers on top. Spoon some sauce over before returning to broiler.

5. Turn skewers every 2 to 3 minutes, basting scallops with a little of the sauce. Scallops will be cooked in 6 to 8 minutes. The outside will be dark brown (but not burnt), while inside flesh will still be succulent.

6. Remove skewers from heat and arrange on plate while vegetables are cooking an extra minute or so. Serve hot.

2 SERVINGS (1 SERVING = 4 OUNCES SCALLOPS AND ½ CUP VEGETABLES)

Tofu Salad

DAY 5

4 ounces fresh tofu (bean curd), cut into ½″ cubes
1 cup shredded carrots
½ cup thinly sliced cucumbers
1 recipe Sesame Dressing (page 284)
Bed of Chinese cabbage (unlimited)
Garnish: 2 tomato wedges and sliced cucumber
(unlimited); toasted sesame seeds (page 162)

1. If preferred, the bean curd can first be parboiled for 1 to 2 minutes and the carrots for 2 to 3 minutes by cooking them in lightly salted boiling water. Set aside until cool.

2. Otherwise, just place the cut vegetables in a deep bowl. Meanwhile, mix together the ingredients for the dressing. Pour the dressing over salad and sprinkle on some toasted sesame seeds. Toss lightly to coat all the ingredients.

3. Serve on a bed of Chinese cabbage. Garnish with tomato and cucumber. Serve at room temperature.

2 SERVINGS (1 SERVING = 2 OUNCES TOFU AND ½ CUP VEGETABLES)

Mixed Grill Yakitori

DAY 5

4 ounces chicken, boned, skinned, cut into 1″ pieces
4 ounces medium shrimp, shelled and deveined
2 scallions, cut into 2″ pieces
⅓ cup sectioned red peppers
⅓ cup sliced zucchini
⅓ cup halved mushrooms
1 recipe Yakitori Sauce (page 283)
4 bamboo skewers

Follow recipe for Chicken Yakitori with Vegetables (Day 3), separating shrimp and vegetables and chicken and vegetables on different skewers, since the cooking times can vary.

2 SERVINGS (1 SERVING = 4 OUNCES TOTAL CHICKEN AND SHRIMP AND ½ CUP VEGETABLES)

Noodles with Broth

DAY 6

2½ ounces dried noodles (udon—Japanese wheat noodles, or soba—Japanese buckwheat noodles)
4 ounces Cooked Chicken Breast (see page 237), skinned, boned and shredded
2 tablespoons finely chopped scallions

BROTH
2 cups dashi (chicken bouillon)
1 tablespoon soy sauce
½ tablespoon water

1. Heat the ingredients for the noodle broth in a saucepan.

2. Cook noodles according to directions on package. Drain in a colander and rinse well under cold water to remove surface starch. Reheat noodles by running hot water over them in colander.

3. Add cooked chicken to hot broth. Place ½ cup hot noodles in two bowls. Pour 1 cup of broth into each bowl with the noodles. Garnish with chopped scallions. Serve hot.

2 SERVINGS (1 SERVING = 2 OUNCES CHICKEN, ½ CUP NOODLES, 1 CUP BROTH)

Fish Teriyaki

DAY 6

1 *pound fresh swordfish steak (fresh tuna or salmon may be substituted)*
½ *cup Teriyaki Sauce (page 277)*
⅔ *cup sectioned red peppers*
⅔ *cup sliced zucchini*
⅔ *cup halved mushrooms*
Garnish: ginger root, cut into slivers

Use recipe for Chicken Teriyaki (Day 1) except that fish will cook in approximately 6 minutes. (The fish is done when it flakes apart with a fork.)

4 SERVINGS (1 SERVING = 4 OUNCES FISH, ½ CUP VEGETABLES)

Baked Fish with Mushrooms in a Package

DAY 7

2 *sheets aluminum foil, slightly larger than 6″ x 10″*
4 *sheets 6″ x 10″ parchment paper*
½ *teaspoon vegetable oil*
½ *pound flounder fillet*
Salt and freshly ground pepper to taste
2 *teaspoons sake*
4 *large mushrooms, sliced thin lengthwise*
Garnish: radish or thin slice of tomato and lemon wedge

1. Preheat oven to 325° F.
2. Spread sheet of foil and then place two pieces of parchment paper on top. Soak a kitchen paper towel in oil and slide between and on top of paper.

3. Cut fish fillet in two and place in center of sheet of aluminum foil. Season each piece with dash of salt and ground pepper. Spoon over 1 teaspoon sake on each and top with mushrooms.

4. Pull up sides of paper to form package and then twist foil to encase package. Place packages on baking sheet in oven and cook for 15 to 20 minutes, opening foil before serving to allow steam to escape.

5. Serve hot, in package, with lemon wedge and either a cut radish or thin slice of tomato for color.

NOTE: This recipe may be used with bay scallops (4 ounces per serving), in which case cooking time will be 3 to 4 minutes longer; or with shrimp (4 ounces per serving), in which case they should be deveined first and then cooked for 20 to 25 minutes or until tinged with pink.

2 SERVINGS (1 SERVING = 4 OUNCES)

Chinese Recipes

Peking Salad

DAYS 1, 3–7

Add one of the following for the corresponding day in the diet:

Day 1   4 *ounces Cooked Chicken Breast (page 237), shredded*
Day 3   4 *ounces frozen or canned baby shrimp*
Day 4   4 *ounces bean curd cake, shredded*
Day 5   1 *cup fresh, cooked salmon, or canned*
Day 6   1 *cup fresh, cooked crabmeat, or canned*
Day 7   1 *cup canned tuna*

and

½ cup fresh beansprouts
¼ cup bamboo shoots (canned), drained and rinsed
¼ cup thinly sliced, canned or fresh water chestnuts, drained and rinsed
Celery cabbage, finely shredded (unlimited)

PEKING SALAD DRESSING
2 tablespoons light soy sauce, or 1½ tablespoons dark sauce and ½ tablespoon water
5 tablespoons (2 lemons) freshly squeezed lemon juice
1 teaspoon freshly grated ginger with juice
Clove garlic, smashed

1. Blanch the beansprouts by pouring boiling water over them. Immediately drain. Cover with cool water and drain again.

290

2. To make dressing, mix ingredients in salad dressing shaker, or any screw-top jar. Shake well. Chill for at least 15 minutes before serving. (Extra dressing may be kept in refrigerator for several days.)

3. Place remaining salad ingredients in bowl and drizzle dressing over, as desired.

4. Toss lightly to coat. Serve at room temperature or chill.

2 SERVINGS (1 SERVING = 2 OUNCES CHICKEN, SHRIMP, BEAN CURD, SALMON, CRABMEAT OR TUNA; ½ CUP VEGETABLES)

Steamed Sea Bass or Red Snapper

DAYS 1 AND 5

1½ pounds whole sea bass or red snapper (cleaned and scaled), or 1 pound fillets
1" chunk ginger root, peeled and cut into pieces, plus 3 thin, round slices of peeled ginger root
2 tablespoons fermented black beans, rinsed before using
2 cloves garlic, finely chopped
2 whole scallions, shredded
2 tablespoons soy sauce
2 tablespoons dry white wine or rice wine

1. Place cleaned fish on heatproof platter and squeeze (over fish) chunks of ginger root in garlic press to extract juice.

2. Rinse black beans and mix with chopped garlic; scatter this mixture, with shredded scallions, soy sauce and wine over fish. Top with ginger slices.

3. To cook, fill a large, metal baking pan halfway with water and place over direct heat on top of stove. Place a trivet in the center and set fish platter on this to steam-cook. Cover the top of baking pan with aluminum foil and crimp edges to seal

291

tight. Turn up heat until water is boiling, and then lower and steam until fish is cooked. (Fillets take from 5 to 10 minutes and a small whole fish cooks in approximately 15 minutes.) Use chopsticks to check that fish is flaky and white.

4. Remove ginger slices and immediately serve directly from platter.

NOTE: The Chinese also eat this dish without the black bean sauce; so if you can't find this ingredient, don't despair. This dish can be made without the black bean flavoring.

4 SERVINGS (1 SERVING = 4 OUNCES)

Stir-Fry Broccoli, Carrots or String Beans
DAYS 1, 2 AND 5

1 tablespoon chicken or vegetable stock
1 clove garlic, crushed
1 cup broccoli (stems cut into 1" pieces and flowerettes into 2" pieces), or 1 cup string beans, cut into 1" pieces, or 1 cup shredded carrots
1 teaspoon soy sauce
Garnish: ½ teaspoon toasted sesame seeds (page 162) (optional)

1. Heat chicken or vegetable stock in nonstick wok or pan over medium heat. Add garlic and cook for 30 seconds, stir-frying.

2. Add vegetables and rapidly stir-fry over high heat for 2 or 3 minutes or until tender but still crunchy. If vegetables stick or liquid evaporates, add more stock.

3. Stir in soy sauce. Serve hot, sprinkled with sesame seeds.

2 SERVINGS (1 SERVING = ½ CUP)

Vermicelli Soup

DAY 2

3½-ounce package cellophane (vermicelli) noodles
2 cups chicken broth
1 cup shredded bokchoy or celery cabbage
½ cup shredded cooked chicken (page 238)
Garnish: 1 tablespoon chopped scallion

1. Soak noodles in hot water 15 minutes to soften. Drain and chop into 4″ lengths.
2. Bring broth to boil in saucepan. Add greens and reduce heat to simmer. Cook for 2 to 3 minutes, until softened.
3. Add noodles and cook for 1 minute more. Add chicken and cook an additional minute over medium heat.
4. Remove from heat and sprinkle scallions on top to garnish.

2 SERVINGS (1 SERVING = 2 OUNCES CHICKEN, ½ CUP COOKED NOODLES, 1 CUP BROTH)

Chinese Vegetable Salad

DAYS 2 AND 4

½ cup peeled, diagonally cut carrots
½ cup diagonally cut zucchini
3½ tablespoons Peking Salad Dressing (page 290)
Celery cabbage, diagonally cut (unlimited)
Garnish: cucumber (Chinese, English or regular), peeled
  and diagonally cut (unlimited)

1. Parboil carrots for 2 to 3 minutes and zucchini for 1 minute. The vegetables should be crisp but tender. Cool.

2. Mix together cooked carrots and zucchini with the dressing. Toss to coat evenly. Let stand at room temperature 1 to 2 hours. Serve on a bed of celery cabbage with sliced cucumber.

2 SERVINGS (1 SERVING = ½ CUP)

Steamed Chicken

DAY 2

8 ounces chicken breasts, boned and skinned
Salt and freshly ground pepper to taste
½-inch chunk fresh ginger root
1 tablespoon fermented black beans (optional), rinsed
*   before using*
½–1 clove garlic, sliced
2 whole scallions, cut in 2-inch pieces and finely
*   shredded*
2 thin diagonal slices fresh ginger root, peeled and
*   shredded*
1 tablespoon thin or light soy sauce
1 tablespoon rice wine or dry sherry

1. Cut the chicken into large chunks. Arrange the pieces on a heatproof plate and season with salt and pepper. Squeeze the chunk of ginger root in a garlic press to extract the juice, over the chicken. Mix the rinsed fermented black beans with the garlic slices and scatter this mixture, along with the shredded scallion and ginger, on top. Pour on the soy sauce and rice wine or sherry.

2. To cook, fill a wok about a third of the way with water and place over direct heat on top of stove and bring to a boil. Place a wire trivet in the bottom of a wok to suspend the heatproof plate over boiling water. Cover the wok with its lid to seal tight. Turn up the heat until boiling, and then lower until chicken is cooked—about 15 to 20 minutes. The chicken should feel firm but not mushy when pressed.

3. Serve immediately with the sauce spooned over the chicken.

2 SERVINGS (1 SERVING = 4 OUNCES)

Spicy Cucumber Salad

DAYS 2 AND 7

3 small Kirby pickling cucumbers
Pinch of salt
3½ tablespoons Peking Salad Dressing (page 290)
1–2 drops hot pepper sauce

1. Prepare cucumbers by washing thoroughly and slicing thin. Place cucumbers in bowl and sprinkle with salt.
2. Mix together the Peking Salad Dressing and a few drops of hot pepper sauce.
3. Pour dressing over the cucumbers. Let stand for 15 minutes. Serve, or chill for 15 to 30 minutes before serving.

2 SERVINGS (UNLIMITED, SERVINGS ARE MERELY A GUIDE)

Stir-Fry Chicken with Asparagus

DAY 3

8 ounces chicken breasts, skinned, boned and cut into 1″ pieces
1 cup asparagus, diagonally sliced in 1″ pieces

MARINADE
1 cup chicken broth
2 tablespoons dry white wine or rice wine
2 cloves garlic, smashed
1 teaspoon grated fresh ginger
1 tablespoon soy sauce

1. Combine marinade ingredients and add chicken. Mix and let stand 10 to 15 minutes.

2. Put 1 tablespoon of marinade into nonstick wok or sauté pan and heat until almost boiling. Add asparagus and stir-fry for 2 minutes over high heat or until tender but still crisp. (Add more chicken broth if necessary.) Remove asparagus from wok with slotted spoon.

3. Bring the rest of the marinade to a boil and add the chicken. Stir-fry, cover, and let cook for 6 to 8 minutes at medium heat. Chicken should be white throughout. Remove chicken from wok, leaving liquid.

4. Reduce sauce to thick glaze of only 3 to 4 tablespoons, then return vegetables and chicken and stir-fry for 30 seconds over high heat. Serve hot.

2 SERVINGS (1 SERVING = 4 OUNCES CHICKEN, ½ CUP VEGETABLES)

Stir-Fry Shrimp with Snow Peas
DAY 4

½ *pound shrimp, shelled and deveined*
1 *tablespoon coarse salt*
1–2 *tablespoons fish or chicken broth*
1 *cup snow peas, trimmed at ends*
1 *teaspoon finely chopped scallion*
Pinch dried red pepper (optional)

MARINADE
4 *teaspoons dry vermouth or sherry*
1½ *teaspoons soy sauce*
1 *clove garlic, crushed*
1 *teaspoon finely minced ginger*

1. Mix together shrimp with 1 teaspoon coarse salt until shrimp are well coated. Let stand 1 minute. Rinse and drain shrimp. Repeat this procedure, mixing another teaspoon of salt

with shrimp, rinsing and draining two more times. Dry shrimp on paper towels. (This gives shrimp a crisp texture, and can be omitted if shrimp is very fresh.)

2. Prepare marinade by mixing ingredients in a bowl. Add shrimp, toss to coat and marinate for 20 to 30 minutes.

3. Heat 1 tablespoon broth in a nonstick wok or skillet until broth begins to boil. Stir-fry shrimp on high heat for 1 to 2 minutes, or until they begin to tinge pink. Remove shrimp with slotted spoon.

4. Add more broth to pan and stir-fry peapods over high heat for approximately 1 minute.

5. Return shrimp to the pan, add scallion and, if desired, dried red pepper. Stir-fry for 2 to 3 minutes, until shrimp is done. If broth is boiling away, then add ½ to 1 teaspoon water. Serve hot.

2 SERVINGS (1 SERVING = 4 OUNCES SHRIMP, ½ CUP VEGETABLES)

Stir-Fry Scallops with Mushrooms and Red Pepper

DAY 6

½ *pound bay scallops or sea scallops, halved*
½ *cup sliced mushrooms or dried Chinese black mushrooms*
½ *cup shredded red pepper*
1 *recipe Marinade (page 296)*

1. Follow recipe for Stir-Fry Shrimp with Snow Peas (Day 4) but eliminate Step 1, soaking the seafood in salt water.

2. If using dried Chinese mushrooms, they have to be soaked before using. Place them in a bowl large enough for them to double in size as they are soaking. Add boiling water to cover. When the mushrooms are soft (20 to 30 minutes), remove from water, leaving behind the sand and grit that has remained

in bottom of bowl. Squeeze the mushrooms dry to remove excess water. Cut off the tough stems and slice them.

3. Scallops usually require a shorter time to stir-fry, so in Step 5, cook about 1 to 2 minutes, depending on scallops' size.

2 SERVINGS (1 SERVING = 4 OUNCES SCALLOPS, ½ CUP VEGETABLES)

Stir-Fry Chicken or Beef with Broccoli

DAY 7

8 *ounces chicken breasts, skinned, boned and cut into 1"*
    pieces, or 8 ounces flank steak, membrane peeled, or
    boneless sirloin (fat removed), thinly sliced against the
    grain into pieces 2" long
1 *cup broccoli, stems cut into 1" pieces, flowerettes into*
    2" pieces

MARINADE
1 *cup chicken or beef broth*
1 *tablespoon dry white wine or rice wine*
2 *cloves garlic, crushed*
1 *teaspoon grated fresh ginger*
1 *tablespoon soy sauce*

1. Combine marinade ingredients and add chicken or beef; mix and let stand 10 to 15 minutes.

2. Put 1 tablespoon marinade into nonstick wok or sauté pan and heat until almost boiling. Add broccoli stems. Stir-fry for 1 minute over high heat and then add flowerettes. Cook for 3 to 4 minutes or until tender but crisp. Remove broccoli from wok.

3. Bring the rest of the marinade to a boil and add chicken or beef. Stir-fry, cover and let cook for 6 to 8 minutes at medium heat. Chicken should be white throughout; beef should be brown. Remove chicken (or beef) from wok, leaving liquid.

4. Reduce sauce to thick glaze of only 3 to 4 table-spoons, then return vegetables and chicken (or beef) and stir-fry for 30 seconds more over high heat. Serve hot.

2 SERVINGS (1 SERVING = 4 OUNCES CHICKEN OR BEEF, ½ CUP VEGETABLE)

Greek Recipes

Greek Salad I, II, III

DAYS 1, 2, 6, 7

GREEK SALAD I
Romaine, escarole, chicory or other lettuce, torn into
    bite-size pieces (unlimited)
Radishes, sliced (unlimited)
Cucumber, sliced (unlimited)
½ cup tomato wedges
¼ cup sliced red onion
¼ cup sliced green pepper (strips or rings)
4 ounces feta cheese
Greek Salad Dressing

GREEK SALAD II
Use all the above ingredients except the feta.

GREEK SALAD III
Use only the salad greens, radishes, cucumber and
    dressing of Greek Salad I.

GREEK SALAD DRESSING
1 clove garlic, peeled and crushed
½ cup lemon juice or wine vinegar
Pinch of oregano
Pinch of mint (fresh or dried)
Salt and freshly ground pepper
(Yields ½ cup)

1. Prepare the salad ingredients and place in a bowl.
2. To prepare dressing, combine all ingredients ex-

cept salt and pepper in a screw-top jar. Shake well. Add salt and pepper to taste. Shake again; refrigerate until used.

3. Pour the dressing on the salad just before serving and toss gently.

2 SERVINGS (1 SERVING = 2 OUNCES FETA AND ½ CUP TOTAL VEGETABLES FOR SALAD I, AND ½ CUP TOTAL VEGETABLES FOR SALAD II; SALAD III IS UN-LIMITED)

Shrimp Mykonos

DAY 1

1½ tablespoons finely chopped onion
1 clove garlic, crushed
Chicken stock or water (optional)
¼ cup finely chopped parsley
1 teaspoon finely chopped dill
⅛ teaspoon dry mustard
1 cup chopped, peeled fresh or canned tomatoes
½ cup Light Tomato Sauce (page 262)
½ pound medium shrimp, peeled and deveined
2 ounces feta cheese or cubed mozzarella

1. Preheat oven to 425° F.
2. Sauté onion and garlic in nonstick skillet until golden, adding a small amount of stock or water if necessary.
3. Add parsley and dill. Stir in mustard. Add tomatoes and Light Tomato Sauce and cook 2 minutes.
4. Rinse and drain the shrimp. Add them to the sauce and cook 1 minute.
5. Pour the mixture into a nonstick casserole and top with the cheese. Bake 10 to 15 minutes, until the cheese is melted. Serve immediately.

2 SERVINGS (1 SERVING = 4 OUNCES)

Saffron Rice

DAYS 1–3, 6–7

½ cup white rice
¾ cup water, chicken or beef stock
Pinch of saffron

1. Combine ingredients in a saucepan.
2. Bring mixture to a boil, stir once, cover and cook on low heat until done, about 17 minutes.

2 SERVINGS (1 SERVING = ½ CUP)

Eggplant Salad

DAY 1

1 (approximately ½ pound) firm medium eggplant
1 small red onion, grated
1 cucumber, peeled and sliced
1 clove garlic, crushed
2 medium tomatoes, peeled, seeded and chopped into
  small pieces
2 tablespoons lemon juice
Salt and freshly ground pepper to taste
Garnish: 4 green or red pepper rings

1. Preheat oven to 350° F.
2. Prick the skin of the eggplant in several places with a fork. Place on a baking sheet. Bake in the oven for 1 hour or until soft. The skin will shrivel and turn black (which in turn gives a smoky flavor to the salad). Remove and let cool slightly.
3. Peel the eggplant when it is still hot (but cool enough to handle) and chop the pulp into small pieces. Place in a bowl. Add the other ingredients. Mix gently.
4. Serve warm or refrigerate for 1 to 2 hours. Garnish with green or red pepper rings.

2 SERVINGS (1 SERVING = ½ CUP)

Grilled Feta Sandwich

DAY 2

4 ounces feta cheese, crumbled
2 whole-wheat pita breads, each split open to form a
    pocket
Dash of oregano

1. Divide the feta cheese in half and stuff the cheese
into each of the pockets. Sprinkle with oregano.
2. Grill under broiler until the cheese melts. Serve
hot.

2 SERVINGS (1 SERVING = 1 PITA)

Baked Chicken with Lemon and Herbs

DAY 2

1 clove garlic, chopped
1 teaspoon fresh or ½ teaspoon dried of any of the
    following herbs, thyme, rosemary, basil, or ¼ teaspoon
    dried ground cumin
½ teaspoon kosher salt
Freshly ground pepper
12 ounces chicken breast, skinned, boned and cut into
    4 pieces
1½–2 tablespoons lemon juice
½–1 cup chicken stock

1. Preheat oven to 350° F.
2. Crush the garlic with the herbs or cumin and salt
and ground pepper, using the side of a knife, until all the salt is
absorbed into garlic.
3. Line baking pan with aluminum foil and arrange

303

pieces of chicken. Rub garlic mixture into the chicken and sprinkle it with lemon juice and half the stock.

4. Bake for 15 minutes, basting with some of the chicken stock. Turn and cook 15 to 20 minutes more, while continuing to baste with the remaining stock. Test for doneness with fork or toothpick—juices should run clear.

5. Serve the chicken hot and chill the remaining for lunch the following day.

4 SERVINGS: 2 DINNER (4 OUNCES EACH) AND 2 LUNCH (2 OUNCES EACH)

Steamed Spinach, Sliced Raw Tomatoes or Steamed Zucchini with Dill and Lemon

DAYS 2, 4 AND 6

1 cup steamed (hot) spinach (page 238), or 1 cup sliced raw tomatoes, or 1 cup sliced steamed (hot) zucchini (page 238)
1 tablespoon finely chopped fresh dill
2 tablespoons freshly squeezed lemon juice
1 clove garlic, smashed
Salt and freshly ground pepper

1. Mix together the dill, lemon juice and garlic and add salt and pepper to taste.

2. Spoon mixture over the hot spinach, raw tomatoes or hot zucchini and serve immediately.

NOTE: For the Steamed Carrots with Dill and Lemon (Jewish Menu, Days 4 and 7) use 1 cup steamed (hot) carrots (page 238) and follow the rest of the above recipe.

2 SERVINGS (1 SERVING = ½ CUP)

Chicken or Tuna Salad

DAYS 3 AND 4

4 ounces Cooked Chicken Breast (page 237), or 1 cup
    canned tuna fish
Romaine, escarole, chicory or other lettuce, torn into
    bite-size pieces (unlimited)
Radishes, sliced (unlimited)
Cucumber, sliced (unlimited)
½ cup tomato wedges
¼ cup sliced red onion
¼ cup sliced green pepper (strips or rings)
Greek Salad Dressing (unlimited) (page 300)

1. Cut the chicken breast into small pieces, or flake
apart tuna.
2. Place in a bowl with the other ingredients. Pour on
the dressing. Gently toss to coat evenly. Serve.

**2 SERVINGS (1 SERVING = 2 OUNCES CHICKEN OR
½ CUP TUNA, ½ CUP VEGETABLES)**

Mediterranean Fish Stew

DAY 3

½ pound codfish fillets
Salt and freshly ground pepper to taste
1–2 tablespoons freshly squeezed lemon juice
¼ cup sliced onion
1 clove garlic, crushed
1 small green pepper, seeded, deribbed and cut into rings
¼ cup chopped fresh parsley
Chicken stock or water (optional)
2 tomatoes, sliced, or 1 cup canned whole plum tomatoes
½ cup hot water

¼ cup dry white wine
1 tablespoon ouzo (anise-flavored Greek liqueur) or
  Pernod

1. Wipe fillets with damp cloth. Cut into chunks. Season with salt and pepper and lemon juice.

2. Heat nonstick skillet; add onion, garlic, pepper and parsley. Add stock or water to keep ingredients from burning. Discard garlic, using a fork or spoon.

3. Add tomatoes, hot water, wine and ouzo or Pernod. Bring just to boiling point; reduce heat.

4. Add the fish and simmer, covered, until fish is done, about 10 minutes. Serve hot.

2 SERVINGS (1 SERVING = 4 OUNCES)

Cucumber and Yogurt Salad

DAYS 3 AND 5

2 medium-size cucumbers, peeled, seeded, quartered
  lengthwise and thinly sliced
1 clove garlic, crushed
Salt and freshly ground pepper to taste
½ teaspoon fresh or ¼ teaspoon dried mint
½ cup plain low-fat yogurt

1. Mix the cucumber slices and garlic together. Place the cucumber slices in layers in a small bowl. Sprinkle each layer lightly with salt. Let stand for 30 minutes. Squeeze the cucumbers to drain off any excess liquid.

2. Season with pepper and sprinkle or crumble the mint over the cucumbers. Beat the yogurt until smooth and pour it over the salad. Mix, then chill for 2 to 3 hours. Serve cold.

2 SERVINGS (1 SERVING = ½ CUP)

Baked Lamb Shanks with New Potatoes

DAY 4

2 *lamb shanks (with ½ pound meat)*
1 *clove garlic, finely minced*
Salt and freshly ground pepper to taste
1 *small carrot, julienned*
½ *cup thinly sliced onion*
1 *rib celery, thinly sliced lengthwise and cut into*
   2" pieces
1 *bay leaf, crumbled*
½ *teaspoon oregano*
¼ *teaspoon dried thyme*
1 *cup sliced plum tomatoes*
4 *new potatoes, peeled*

1. Preheat oven to 350° F.

2. Cut fat from under shank, score top skin with sharp knife and rub with garlic. Season with salt and pepper.

3. Fill the bottom of a roasting pan with the carrot, onion, celery and bay leaf. Add the lamb shanks; season with oregano and thyme. Add tomatoes. Cover tightly and bake 2 to 2½ hours, depending on the size of the shanks.

4. During the last hour of cooking uncover the roasting pan and add the potatoes. Continue cooking, uncovered, basting the potatoes and meat with cooked vegetables in the pan.

5. Serve the shanks with the potatoes and the cooked vegetables separately.

2 SERVINGS (1 SERVING = 4 OUNCES LAMB, OFF THE BONE, AND 2 POTATOES)

Greek Fruit Salad

DAY 4

1 *small navel orange*
½ cup watermelon chunks (reserve any juice)
6 green seedless grapes
Garnish: 2 mint leaves

1. Peel the orange and remove the white membrane (which is quite bitter). Slice the orange crosswise into thin slices, saving as much juice as possible. Remove any pits.

2. Add the melon chunks and orange slices and their juice to a bowl. Scatter the grapes with the other fruit and gently toss.

3. Serve cold or at room temperature in glass goblets or wineglasses. Garnish with a mint leaf.

2 SERVINGS (1 SERVING = ½ CUP)

Shrimp and Tomato Salad

DAY 5

4 ounces shrimp, shelled and deveined then boiled and
  chilled
1 cup tomato wedges
Cucumber, thinly sliced (unlimited)
Greek Salad Dressing (page 300)
Bed of romaine or Boston lettuce (unlimited)
Garnish: sliced radishes (unlimited)

1. Mix the shrimp, tomato wedges and cucumber together first.

2. Pour on dressing to taste and mix. Serve on a bed of lettuce, garnished with sliced radishes.

2 SERVINGS (1 SERVING = 2 OUNCES SHRIMP, ½ CUP TOMATOES)

308

Stuffed Eggplant

DAY 5

2 *small or 1 medium eggplant (approximately 1 pound)*
¼ cup finely chopped onion
Veal, chicken stock or water (optional)
2 cloves garlic, mashed
8 ounces ground veal
1 canned whole tomato, chopped
1 cup cooked White Rice (page 278) or Saffron Rice (page 302)
½ teaspoon pine nuts (pignoli)
2 tablespoons finely chopped fresh parsley
1 teaspoon finely chopped fresh dill
¼ teaspoon fresh or dried marjoram or mint
⅛–¼ teaspoon grated nutmeg or allspice
Salt and freshly ground pepper to taste
½ cup veal or chicken stock
Garnish: chopped parsley or dill

1. Preheat oven to 350° F.

2. Wash skin of eggplant(s), halve eggplants lengthwise and carefully scoop out the pulp, leaving a shell ¼" thick. Chop pulp finely.

3. Sauté onion slowly in a nonstick skillet until soft, adding water or stock if necessary, to prevent sticking. Add garlic and ground veal and sauté until browned. Then cook eggplant pulp and chopped tomato with it for 5 minutes. Add rice, pine nuts, parsley, dill, marjoram or mint and then season with nutmeg or allspice and salt and pepper to taste. Cook gently for 5 more minutes.

4. Spoon mixture into eggplant shells. Arrange them in a shallow baking dish. Pour in enough water to come halfway up their sides.

5. Bake in oven for 45 minutes, or until eggplant shells are cooked through and are soft but have not lost their shape. Pour over 2 tablespoons of the veal or chicken stock on

each of the eggplant shells 15 minutes before they are done. Garnish with chopped parsley or dill. Serve hot.

2 SERVINGS (1 SERVING = 1 [½ POUND] EGGPLANT)

Veal Kebabs

DAY 6

3 ounces ground veal
1 tablespoon grated onion
1 teaspoon lemon juice
Pinch of marjoram
Pinch of salt and freshly ground pepper
2 ½" (2 ounce) cubes of feta cheese
2 whole-wheat pita bread, slit in half to form a pocket

1. Mix with the ground veal: onion, lemon juice, pinch of marjoram and salt and pepper.
2. Shape into 2 patties and insert 1 cube of feta cheese into each patty.
3. Broil on each side until the meat is browned outside and cheese is melted inside.
4. Serve encased in a pocket of pita bread.

2 SERVINGS (1 SERVING = 1 PATTY)

Fish Plaki

DAY 6

1½–1¾ pounds red snapper or any other firm flesh fish,
cleaned and scaled but with head and tail intact
½ teaspoon salt
½ teaspoon oregano
Freshly ground pepper

¼ cup chopped scallion
⅛ cup finely chopped parsley, preferably flat
½ teaspoon finely chopped garlic
2 small or 1 medium tomato, cut into ½" slices
2 tablespoons of fine fresh bread crumbs or cracker crumbs
    (made from salt-free soda crackers pulverized by hand
    or electric blender)
1 small lemon, thinly sliced
1 small onion, thinly sliced
2 tablespoons of dry white wine or vermouth
Garnish: sprigs of parsley

1. Preheat oven to 350° F.

2. Wash and dry the fish. Score diagonally across one of its sides with three ½"-deep gashes spaced 2" apart. Place it in a nonstick or regular baking dish (i.e., ceramic).

3. Combine salt, oregano and pepper and press it into the gashes.

4. Mix together the scallion, parsley and garlic and scatter mixture on fish. Arrange the tomato slices in two parallel lines lengthwise down the fish. Sprinkle the bread or cracker crumbs on top of tomato slices. Alternate slices of lemon and onion on top of and in the middle of the two rows of tomatoes.

5. Bake for 20 to 30 minutes or until done. Fifteen minutes into the cooking time add the wine over the fish. The fish should still feel firm when pressed with your fingers. Do not overcook.

6. Garnish with parsley sprigs and serve.

4 SERVINGS (1 SERVING = 4 OUNCES)

Dolmitas
(Stuffed Grape Leaves)

DAY 7

2 tablespoons finely chopped onion
¼–¾ cup veal or chicken stock or water
4 ounces ground veal
1 clove garlic, mashed
⅛ teaspoon allspice
⅛ teaspoon mint
1 tablespoon finely chopped fresh parsley
1 teaspoon finely chopped fresh dill
1 cup cooked White Rice (page 278)
Salt and freshly ground pepper to taste
8 (approximately 4 ounces) grape leaves, packed in brine
Juice of ½ lemon
½ cup tomato juice (or veal or chicken stock)
·Garnish: parsley sprigs and lemon wedges

1. Sauté onion slowly in nonstick pan until soft, adding stock or water if necessary to prevent sticking or burning. Then sauté veal with garlic and herbs until browned. Add rice and season with salt and pepper to taste. Cook gently for 5 more minutes, and add the additional ¼ cup of veal or chicken stock.

2. Rinse preserved grape leaves carefully (as they tear easily) and thoroughly in hot water to remove all brine. Dry them on paper towel.

3. Put about 1 tablespoon of meat stuffing on each leaf stem end, fold over end and sides. Roll leaf up from stem end.

4. Place the rolled leaves carefully in a nonstick skillet or regular skillet rolled sides down. Squeeze on the lemon juice. Add ¼ cup of the tomato juice or stock (enough to come halfway up the sides of dolmitas). Place a heatproof plate on top of dolmitas.

5. Simmer gently for 20 to 30 minutes. As juice or

stock evaporates, add the remaining ¼ cup of the liquid. Cool, and refrigerate at least 2 hours before serving. Garnish with parsley and lemon wedges.

2 SERVINGS (1 SERVING = 4 STUFFED GRAPE LEAVES)

Chilled Cucumber-Yogurt Soup

DAY 7

½ cup plain low-fat yogurt
½ cup skim milk
1 medium cucumber, peeled, halved, seeded and grated
1 teaspoon white vinegar
1 teaspoon finely grated onion
1 teaspoon finely cut fresh mint, or ½ teaspoon dried mint
½ teaspoon finely chopped fresh dill
Pinch of salt and freshly ground pepper
Garnish: mint leaves and cucumber, thinly sliced (unlimited)

1. Mix yogurt and skim milk in a bowl with wire whisk until blended and completely smooth.
2. Beat in gently cucumber, vinegar, onion, mint, dill and salt until mixed. Alternatively, all these ingredients can be blended in electric blender or food processor. Season with freshly ground pepper and refrigerate 2 hours.
3. Serve chilled, garnished with mint leaf and thinly sliced cucumber.

2 SERVINGS (1 SERVING = 1 CUP)

Greek-Style Chicken

DAY 7

8 ounces chicken breasts, skinned, boned
Salt and freshly ground pepper to taste
1 clove garlic, crushed
1 cup fresh or canned Italian plum tomatoes
¼ bay leaf
¼ teaspoon dried thyme
2 small white onions, peeled and sliced
4 wafer-thin lemon slices
½ cup water (optional)
Garnish: 2 tablespoons finely chopped parsley

1. Season chicken breast with salt and pepper and rub with garlic.

2. Put tomatoes, bay leaf, thyme and onions into nonstick pan and cook over medium heat for 10 minutes until onions become transparent.

3. Place chicken breast into pan and put lemon slices on top of chicken.

4. Cover and cook for 25 minutes over moderate heat, stirring occasionally and adding water if necessary. Test meat by piercing with knife or toothpick; when juices run clear, meat is done.

5. Garnish with chopped parsley and serve hot.

NOTE: This dish is sometimes served with mussels. In that case, use 4 ounces of skinned and boned chicken breast and 20 small mussels. Clean, debeard and soak the mussels for 1 to 2 hours in several changes of cold water until most of the sand is gone. Steam them until opened, about 10 minutes. Add these to sauce during last 15 minutes of cooking time.

2 SERVINGS (1 SERVING = 4 OUNCES)

Mexican Recipes

Turkey, Chicken or Monterey Jack Taco

DAYS 1, 4, 6

1 *tortilla*
2 *ounces Cooked Turkey or Chicken Breast (page 237),*
  shredded, or shredded Monterey Jack cheese
½ *cup diced tomato*
Romaine lettuce, shredded (unlimited)
Garnish: 1 onion slice and cucumber, diced (unlimited)
1 *cup Salsa (Sauce) (below)*

1. Heat the tortilla in 200° F. oven until warm, or heat in a nonstick pan.
2. Place the chicken or turkey or cheese, tomato and lettuce on top and douse them with Salsa.
3. Roll up and serve, garnished with onion slice and diced cucumber.

1 SERVING

Salsa
(Sauce)

¼ *cup finely chopped onions*
¼ *cup chicken broth*
½ *cup finely chopped green pepper*
2 *cloves garlic, chopped*
1 *8-ounce can tomato sauce*

2 ounces canned green chiles, diced, or 2 ounces fresh
chiles, seeded, peeled and chopped
1 teaspoon oregano or ground cumin

1. In a skillet, gently sauté onion in 2 tablespoons chicken broth over low heat. Cover pan, but watch and stir to prevent burning. If necessary, add additional chicken stock. Cook for 10 minutes, or until onion becomes transparent.

2. Add green pepper and garlic and cook for 5 minutes. If necessary, additional broth may be added.

3. Pour in any remaining chicken broth, tomato sauce, chiles and oregano. Turn up heat and simmer, covered, for 5 minutes.

4. Put sauce into electric blender until color is consistent, stopping before ingredients are completely liquefied.

5. If necessary, reheat before serving. Any sauce not used may be poured into screw-top jar and kept in refrigerator for several days.

YIELD: 1¼ CUPS

Ensalada I
(Mexican Salad)

Romaine lettuce, shredded (unlimited)
Radishes, sliced (unlimited)
Cucumber, chopped (unlimited)
1 Jalapeño chile pepper (canned or fresh), diced
  (optional)
Chili Salad Dressing

CHILI SALAD DRESSING
¼ cup lime juice (juice of 3 limes)
¾ cup tomato juice
⅛ teaspoon chili powder
1 teaspoon finely chopped fresh coriander leaves, or
  ½ teaspoon dried
(Yields 1 cup)

316

1. To prepare dressing, combine ingredients in a screw-top jar and shake well. Refrigerate until used. Shake jar again before serving.

2. Place salad ingredients in a bowl. Spoon dressing over. Toss gently. Serve.

2 SERVINGS (1 SERVING = UNLIMITED)

Chicken Breasts Picante con Chiles
(Spicy Chicken Breasts with Chiles)

DAY 1

1 3-ounce can green chiles, sliced
8 ounces chicken breasts, skinned and boned
½ cup chopped onion
1 cup Salsa (Sauce) (page 315)
½ medium tomato, thinly sliced
½ ounce white cheddar cheese, grated

1. Preheat oven to 350° F.

2. Cut green chiles into strips, and chicken breasts into 1" pieces.

3. Arrange half the onion on bottom of a nonstick baking pan; place half the pieces of chicken breasts on top and cover with half the slices of chile.

4. Repeat the layers with the rest of ingredients and pour sauce on top.

5. Bake in oven for 20 minutes, then arrange slices of tomato on top and sprinkle with cheese.

6. Bake until chicken is done and the cheese is melted, about 20 more minutes. Serve hot.

2 SERVINGS (1 SERVING = 4 OUNCES)

Mexican Rice

DAYS 1, 2, 4, 6, 7

¼ cup chopped onion
1 clove garlic, peeled and finely chopped
Chicken stock or water (optional)
1 cup white rice
1¾ cups chicken stock
¼ cup canned or fresh tomato puree

1. Sauté onion and garlic gently in nonstick pan until golden brown, adding a small amount of stock or water if necessary. Mix together the onion with the rice.
2. Pour in the chicken stock. Bring the mixture to a boil, cover and cook until rice is done, about 17 minutes. Or bake in a preheated 375° F. oven until done (the liquid is absorbed). Just before serving, stir in the tomato puree and cook until heated through—about 3 minutes. Serve hot.

4 SERVINGS (1 SERVING = ½ CUP)

Ensalada II
(Mexican Salad)

DAYS 1 AND 3

Romaine lettuce, shredded (unlimited)
Radishes, sliced (unlimited)
Cucumber, chopped (unlimited)
½ cup chopped tomato
¼ cup chopped green and red pepper
¼ cup chopped onion
1 Jalapeño chile pepper (canned or fresh), diced
    (optional)
Chili Salad Dressing (unlimited) (page 316)

1. Place salad ingredients in a bowl.
2. Pour on dressing. Toss gently. Serve.

2 SERVINGS (1 SERVING = ½ CUP TOTAL CHOPPED VEGETABLES)

Ensalada III (Mexican Salad) with Tuna or Turkey

DAYS 2 AND 5

½ cup tuna, or 2 ounces Cooked Turkey Breast (page 237), shredded
Romaine lettuce, shredded (unlimited)
Cucumber, chopped (unlimited)
½ cup chopped green and red pepper
½ cup chopped tomato
1 Jalapeño chile pepper (canned or fresh), diced (optional)
Chili Salad Dressing (unlimited) (page 316)

1. Add tuna or turkey to other salad ingredients.
2. Pour on 2 to 4 tablespoons of the salad dressing. Mix well and serve chilled.

2 SERVINGS (1 SERVING = ½ CUP TUNA OR 2 OUNCES TURKEY, ½ CUP TOTAL CHOPPED VEGETABLES)

Veal Chops Veracruz

DAY 2

1–2 cloves garlic, finely minced
½ cup thinly sliced onion
Chicken or veal stock or water (optional)
2 (4 ounces each) rib or shoulder veal chops

319

½–1 teaspoon dry mustard
Salt and freshly ground pepper to taste
¼ cup dry white wine
¼ cup freshly squeezed lemon juice
½ cup green pepper strips

1. Brown garlic and onion in nonstick pan, adding a small amount of veal or chicken stock or water, if necessary. Set mixture aside.

2. Season veal chops with mustard, salt and pepper. Brown on both sides and add wine and lemon juice. Cook over low heat until sauce is reduced and thick. Add onion, garlic and green pepper. Cover pan.

3. Continue to cook over low heat until chops are done. Serve hot with remaining sauce poured over chops.

2 SERVINGS (1 SERVING = 4 OUNCES)

Steamed Zucchini or Chayote with Tomato Sauce

DAYS 2 AND 4

1 cup sliced zucchini or chayote
2 tablespoons tomato puree, heated
Few grains chili powder

1. Steam zucchini or chayote (see page 238) until tender, but still crisp, about 5 minutes for the zucchini and slightly longer for the chayote.

2. Serve hot with tomato puree spooned on top and few grains of chili powder.

2 SERVINGS (1 SERVING = ½ CUP)

Monterey Jack *or* Turkey and Monterey Jack Quesadilla

DAYS 3 AND 7

1 *tortilla*
2 *ounces Monterey Jack cheese, grated, or 1 ounce*
  Cooked Turkey Breast (page 237), shredded, and 1
  ounce Monterey Jack cheese, grated
½ *cup finely chopped green pepper*
¼ *cup finely chopped onion*
Garnish: ¼ cup chopped tomato

1. Place tortilla shell in nonstick pan. Heat until crisp.
2. Fill with ingredients by layering them.
3. Lift half of tortilla with spatula and fold over.
4. Cook on low heat until cheese melts. Serve immediately, garnished with chopped tomato.

NOTE: One or two tablespoons of Salsa (page 315) may be added to the Turkey and Monterey Jack Quesadilla filling to bind it together.

1 SERVING

Lime Chicken

DAY 3

2 (or 1 *pound) whole chicken breasts, skinned and split*
½–1 *tablespoons paprika*
½ *teaspoon salt*
¼ *teaspoon freshly ground pepper*
¾ *cup lime juice (6 limes)*
1 *fresh hot green pepper, seeded and finely diced, or*
  2 *ounces canned chile peppers, diced*

321

1 *cup sliced onion rings*
1 *cup sweet red pepper rings*
Garnish: fresh coriander (optional)

1. Season chicken with paprika, ¼ teaspoon salt, freshly ground pepper.

2. Marinate chicken in half the lime juice and hot pepper, 10–12 hours (overnight) in refrigerator, turning breasts occasionally.

3. Place the chicken breasts under broiler, or on a charcoal grill. Baste with marinade, and turn often, until cooked. Turn oven temperature down to 350° F.

4. Meanwhile, blanch onion rings for 1 minute in boiling water. Heat remaining lime juice and salt and add the onion rings. Cook until tender.

5. Place onion and sweet pepper rings on top of chicken, reheat in oven for 5 minutes.

6. Serve hot and, if desired, garnish with coriander.
NOTE: This dish has to be prepared 1 day in advance.

4 SERVINGS (1 SERVING = 4 OUNCES)

Veal en Salsa (in Sauce)

DAY 4

8 *ounces veal*
Salt and freshly ground pepper to taste
1 *tablespoon oregano*
1¼ *cups Salsa (Sauce) (page 315)*

1. Preheat oven to 350° F.

2. Cut veal into 1″ cubes and place in nonstick baking pan.

3. Season veal with salt, pepper and oregano.

4. Add Salsa and bake in oven until done, 20 to 30 minutes.

2 SERVINGS (1 SERVING = 4 OUNCES)

322

Chicken Enchiladas

DAY 5

14 ounces Cooked Chicken Breast (page 237), diced
2 ounces shredded Monterey Jack cheese
½ cup diced onion
1½ cups Salsa (Sauce) (page 315)
4 tortillas
Garnish: 2 tablespoons chopped scallion

1. Preheat oven to 350° F.
2. Mix the chicken with cheese, diced onion, and ¼ cup of the Salsa. Set aside.
3. Heat remaining Salsa. Dip the tortillas for a few seconds into the simmering sauce to coat them and then remove. Fill each with one-quarter of the chicken-cheese-onion mixture. Roll up and place open side down in shallow baking dish.
4. Pour sauce over enchiladas. Bake in nonstick baking dish for 20 to 25 minutes, or until cheese melts.
5. Garnish with chopped scallion. Serve hot.

4 SERVINGS (1 SERVING = 1 ENCHILADA)

Red Snapper Veracruz

DAY 6

1¼–1½ pounds red snapper
½ teaspoon salt
1 tablespoon lime juice (from ½ lime)
½ cup finely sliced onion
1 small clove garlic, peeled and sliced
2 tablespoons chicken stock
1 8-ounce can whole plum tomatoes
1 bay leaf

½ tablespoon large capers
1 Jalapeño chile, skinned and cut into strips

1. Clean fish, cut into pieces and prick both sides with a fork. Marinate in mixture of salt and lime juice for 2 hours.
2. Preheat oven to 325° F.
3. Sauté onions and garlic in chicken stock over low heat. Cover pan, but watch and stir to prevent burning. If necessary, add additional stock. Cook for 10 minutes, or until onion becomes transparent.
4. Add tomatoes and the rest of ingredients. Cook sauce over high heat to evaporate some of the juice, 2 to 5 minutes.
5. Place fish in nonstick baking dish. Pour sauce over fish and bake, uncovered, for 20 minutes, basting with the sauce. Turn and continue cooking an additional 10 minutes if necessary.

NOTE: Do not use foil-lined pan, as fish and sauce will pick up metallic taste.

4 SERVINGS (1 SERVING = 4 OUNCES)

Pompano en Salsa Verde (in Green Tomato Sauce)

DAY 7

1 pound pompano or sea bass
⅛ teaspoon peppercorns
⅛ teaspoon cumin seeds
⅛–¼ teaspoon salt
Juice of 1 large lime

SALSA VERDE (GREEN TOMATO SAUCE)
1 small clove garlic
¼ green pepper
½ fresh serrano chile (a small, smooth, medium green chile pepper)

324

1 *sprig fresh coriander*
1 *sprig parsley*
2 *scallions*
⅛ *teaspoon oregano*
1 *teaspoon mild white vinegar*
½ *pound green (unripe) tomatoes*
2 *tablespoons water*

1. Clean and scale fish, leaving head and tail intact.

2. Grind spices and add lime juice.

3. Prick fish with a fork and marinate in lime juice and spices for 1 hour.

4. Preheat oven to 300° F.

5. To prepare Salsa Verde, chop all remaining ingredients coarsely and blend them (in blender or food processor) to a smooth sauce.

6. Pour sauce over fish in a nonstick baking dish. Cook fish, uncovered, in the oven for 20 minutes. Turn fish over and continue to bake another 15 to 20 minutes. Baste with sauce.

4 SERVINGS (1 SERVING = 4 OUNCES)

Jewish Recipes

Turkey Cutlets with Cranberry-Fruit Relish

DAY 1

8 ounces turkey breast cutlets, thinly sliced
Salt and freshly ground pepper
2 tablespoons chicken stock

CRANBERRY-FRUIT RELISH
8 ounces fresh cranberries, washed and picked over
1 small ripe tangerine
1 cup unsweetened applesauce, or 1 cup canned
   unsweetened, crushed pineapple, drained
(Yields 2 cups, approximately)

1. To prepare relish, wash, peel and section tangerine, reserving skin. Pull each fruit section apart and remove seeds.
2. Put all ingredients, including tangerine skin, into blender and puree until color is consistent, but sauce still has some texture. Spoon into screw-top jar and chill. (Relish will keep in refrigerator for a week or more and is excellent with all poultry and cold meat.)
3. Preheat broiler to medium/high.
4. Line pan with foil and put in turkey breast slices. Season turkey with salt and pepper and place under broiler for 5 to 8 minutes, until meat turns color. Turn and cook the other side. Spoon chicken stock over meat during last 2 to 3 minutes of cooking time and turn broiler to high. This promotes browning, but should not be allowed to burn.

2 SERVINGS (1 SERVING = 4 OUNCES TURKEY, ½ CUP RELISH)

Coleslaw Salad

DAYS 1, 4 AND 6

1½ cups shredded and chopped red or green cabbage
¼ cup chopped green or red pepper
¼ cup grated carrot
1 tablespoon grated onion (optional)
3 tablespoons chopped fresh dill, or 2 teaspoons caraway
  or celery seeds
3 tablespoons white vinegar or lemon juice
3 tablespoons cold water
Salt and freshly ground pepper to taste

1. Mix all ingredients together well.
2. Let stand in refrigerator for 2 hours or overnight.
(This cabbage salad will keep in the refrigerator for several days.)
Serve cold.

4 SERVINGS (1 SERVING = ½ CUP)

Stuffed Veal Rib Chops

DAY 2

¾ cup finely chopped mushrooms
¼ cup finely chopped onion, or 2 tablespoons finely
  chopped shallots
Veal stock or water (optional)
¼ teaspoon grated nutmeg
Pinch of black pepper
2 4-ounce veal rib chops

1. Squeeze mushrooms in a dish towel, twisting to
remove moisture content. Set mushrooms aside.
2. Cook the onion or shallots slowly until golden in a
nonstick pan, adding a small amount of stock or water if necessary. Add mushrooms, nutmeg and black pepper. Sauté over

327

high heat until moisture from mushrooms is almost completely evaporated.

    3. Cut a large gash in side of each chop to form a pocket. Fill each pocket with mushroom stuffing. Close with thin wooden skewers or toothpicks.

    4. Broil on both sides until done.

2 SERVINGS (1 SERVING = 4 OUNCES)

Kasha (Buckwheat Groats)

DAY 2

1 *cup veal, chicken or beef stock*
½ *cup whole kasha*
1 *shallot, minced*
1 *tablespoon chopped fresh parsley or dill*
Dash of cayenne pepper

    1. Bring stock to a boil in a saucepan.

    2. Add kasha and minced shallot and bring to boil again. Reduce heat, stir well and simmer, uncovered, for precisely 8 minutes (not longer). If necessary, add a few tablespoons more of stock. The kasha is done when all the liquid has been absorbed and each kernel is separate.

    3. Add parsley or dill and pepper, toss well and serve immediately.

2 SERVINGS (1 SERVING = ½ CUP)

Cucumber Salad

DAYS 2, 5 AND 7

3 Kirby pickling cucumbers
¼ cup lemon juice or vinegar
1 tablespoon grated onion
1 tablespoon chopped fresh dill
Salt and freshly ground pepper to taste

1. Wash the cucumbers thoroughly and slice them thinly.
2. Place in a bowl with lemon juice or vinegar, onion and dill. Toss gently. Season with salt and pepper to taste.
3. Let stand either at room temperature or in refrigerator for 30 minutes before serving.

2 SERVINGS (1 SERVING = UNLIMITED)

Baked Apple

DAYS 2 AND 7

4 small baking apples
Dash of cinnamon
1 teaspoon vanilla

1. Preheat oven to 350° F.
2. Core the apples and cut a ½" slice off the top. Place apples in a baking dish.
3. Sprinkle with cinnamon and vanilla.
4. Bake for 15 to 30 minutes, until soft.

4 SERVINGS (1 SERVING = 1 APPLE)

Gefilte Fish

DAY 3

½ pound pike and ½ pound whitefish, cleaned and
   scaled (retain head, tail, skin and bones)
2 onions—1 large, 1 small
1 egg, well beaten
¼ cup cold water
¼ teaspoon each salt and pepper
1 tablespoon matzoh meal
1 carrot, thinly sliced
Salt and freshly ground pepper to taste
Garnish: 2–3 tablespoons chopped fresh parsley, lemon
   wedges and/or horseradish (unlimited)

1. Chop fish and large onion together very finely in a
food processor or blender.
2. In a large bowl add fish and onion mixture, beaten
egg, water, salt, pepper and matzoh meal. Mix well until fluffy.
3. Place head, tail, skin and bones of fish in a large
pan and add water to cover.
4. Add small onion, carrot, salt and pepper. Bring to
a boil. Wet hands before shaping fish mixture into small oval-
shaped balls equal to about 2 tablespoons each. Drop the balls
into the boiling stock. Reduce heat, cover and simmer slowly for
1½ to 2 hours.
5. Cool. Strain the fish stock and reserve the carrot.
6. Refrigerate the fish balls and strained fish stock
(with the carrot) separately, and serve them cold garnished with
the jelled fish stock, chopped parsley, a slice of cooked carrot,
lemon wedges and horseradish.
NOTE: It is best to prepare this dish 1 day in advance.

**6 TO 8 SERVINGS APPROXIMATELY
(1 SERVING = 2 OUNCES OR 2 SMALL BALLS)**

Turkey Loaf

DAYS 3 AND 4

1 *pound ground turkey*
1 *egg white*
2 *tablespoons chopped fresh parsley*
1 *teaspoon lemon juice*
½ *teaspoon thyme*
¼ *teaspoon freshly ground pepper*
1 *clove garlic*
1 *teaspoon kosher (coarse) salt*
Garnish: paprika and bay leaf

1. Preheat oven to 350° F.
2. Combine turkey, egg white, parsley, lemon juice, thyme and pepper.
3. Chop garlic clove fine and then sprinkle with kosher salt. Crush garlic into salt with flat of knife, scraping and crushing until all garlic is absorbed. Blend this into other ingredients and shape mixture into loaf in a nonstick pan.
4. Decorate with bay leaf and swirl of paprika. Bake approximately 1¼ hours. Loaf will shrink from sides and juices run clear.
5. Serve hot with vegetables as entree, or cold, thinly sliced, for following day's lunch.

5 SERVINGS: 3 DINNER (4 OUNCES EACH) AND 2 LUNCH (2 OUNCES EACH)

Cold Pickled Beets

DAYS 3 AND 4

2 cups cold cooked (boiled) beets
½ teaspoon salt
⅛ teaspoon pepper
⅓ cup water
⅓ cup white vinegar
¼ teaspoon caraway seeds, or ¼ cup sliced onion

1. Slice the beets and place in a bowl.
2. Add the salt, pepper, water, vinegar, caraway seeds or sliced onion, and mix well.
3. Chill for 1 to 2 hours and serve.

4 SERVINGS (1 SERVING = ½ CUP)

Unsweetened Applesauce

DAYS 3 AND 6

4 small Delicious (yellow or red) apples
Water
Dash of cinnamon
1 teaspoon vanilla

1. Peel and quarter apples. Place in a saucepan, and partly cover with water.
2. Simmer until tender.
3. Puree the apples through a food mill, strainer or blender.
4. Add a dash of cinnamon and vanilla.
5. Serve hot or cold.
NOTE: You may also combine 1 cup crushed unsweetened pineapple or 1 cup fresh or frozen unsweetened (thawed)

raspberries with the applesauce. In that case, use only 1 cup of applesauce.

4 SERVINGS (1 SERVING = ½ CUP, APPROXIMATELY)

Stuffed Cabbage Rolls

DAY 4

1 head cabbage
1 pound lean ground veal, or ½ pound each lean ground
    veal and lean ground beef
½ cup cooked White Rice (see page 278)
½ cup minced onion
3 tablespoons finely chopped fresh parsley
½ teaspoon dried thyme
Salt and freshly ground pepper to taste
1 6-ounce can tomato paste
1 16-ounce can whole plum tomatoes, coarsely chopped
1½ teaspoons white vinegar or lemon juice
½ carrot, grated
2 bay leaves

1. Preheat oven to 325° F.

2. Cut away the hard center core of the cabbage. Separate the cabbage into individual leaves.

3. Cook 10 to 12 leaves in pot of boiling water for 2 minutes, until tender. Drain in colander, and immediately submerge cabbage leaves in cold water. Drain well on paper towel to remove excess water. Be careful not to tear the leaves.

4. Mix together the veal, rice, onion, parsley, thyme, salt, pepper and 3 tablespoons of tomato paste.

5. Fill 8 cabbage leaves with 3 to 4 tablespoons of meat mixture. Carefully roll up and, if necessary, fasten the rolled side with toothpicks. Place rolled side down in a baking pan.

6. Mix together remaining tomato paste, tomatoes, vinegar, carrot and bay leaves. Pour over the cabbage rolls.

7. Cook, covered, for about 1½ hours. It can also be cooked in a covered Dutch oven by simmering for about 1 hour on top of the stove. If the tomato sauce evaporates, it may be necessary to add some water (up to 1 cup). For both methods, remove the cover during the last 15 minutes of cooking time. If the sauce is not thick after this time, then reduce it in a saucepan.

8. Serve the cabbage rolls hot with the sauce spooned over.

NOTE: This dish benefits in taste if it is cooked 1 day in advance.

4 SERVINGS (1 SERVING = 2 CABBAGE ROLLS— 4 OUNCES VEAL)

Borscht (Beet Soup)

DAY 5

2 *cups shredded beets*
4 *cups chicken stock or water*
¼ *cup minced onion*
1 *teaspoon salt*
¼ *cup lemon juice*
4 *small boiled potatoes*
Garnish: 1 *tablespoon plain low-fat yogurt*

1. Combine first 4 ingredients in a pot and simmer for about 1 hour.

2. Add lemon juice.

3. Chill; serve with boiled potato. Garnish with a tablespoon of yogurt.

4 SERVINGS (1 SERVING = 1 CUP SOUP AND 1 PO- TATO)

Chicken in a Pot

DAY 5

2 (*approximately* 1 *pound*) *whole chicken breasts, split*
6 *cups canned chicken broth*
2 *cups carrots, peeled and cut into* 2" *pieces*
4 *celery ribs, halved*
4 *small boiling onions*
1 *parsnip*
8 *sprigs parsley and/or* 8 *sprigs fresh dill, tied together*
  with string
10 *peppercorns*
Kosher (*coarse*) *salt to taste*
2 *cups cooked noodles*

1. Place the chicken breasts in a deep soup pot and add the chicken broth. Add the carrots, celery, onions, parsnip, parsley and/or dill, peppercorns and salt.

2. Bring to a boil and skim off any fat and scum that form on the surface. Cover and cook at a simmer for 1 hour.

3. Strain the soup, chicken and vegetables into a colander lined with cheesecloth with a bowl placed underneath to catch the liquid. Pour the soup back into the pot and skim off any remaining fat. Reserve only the chicken and carrots. Remove the skin from the chicken.

4. Return the chicken and carrots to the pot. Serve in deep bowls with hot cooked noodles.

4 SERVINGS (1 SERVING = 4 OUNCES CHICKEN, ½ CUP COOKED NOODLES, ½ CUP CARROTS, 1 CUP BROTH)

Chopped Chicken Liver

DAY 6

8 ounces chicken livers
¼ teaspoon salt
½ teaspoon freshly ground pepper
½ medium onion, sliced thin
1 hard-cooked egg white
1–2 tablespoons chicken stock

1. Wash the livers thoroughly in cold water, then sprinkle both sides with salt and pepper. Place livers and sliced onion on a sheet of foil and set under medium broiler until they change color, 10 to 12 minutes. Turn and grill second side the same way. (Alternatively, the onion may first be sautéed slowly in a small amount of chicken stock in a nonstick pan until soft. Then add the liver and cook until just done.)

2. Cool and put onion slices and livers through electric blender or food processor to chop until they are a fine paste. Add white of egg and chop briefly, then add chicken stock and mix until the consistency is smoother (add more, if desired).

3. Pack chopped liver into a small earthenware dish and chill for several hours or until the next day.

NOTE: This dish benefits in taste if prepared 1 day in advance.

4 SERVINGS (1 SERVING = 2 OUNCES)

Baked Fish with Tomato Sauce

DAY 6

1 pound fillet of scrod or halibut
1 8-ounce can tomato sauce
Juice of ½ lemon
Salt and freshly ground pepper to taste
Garnish: chopped fresh parsley

1. Preheat oven to 350° F.

2. Place fish in nonstick pan, add tomato sauce, lemon juice, salt and pepper. Bake for 20 minutes, or until done, basting if necessary.

3. Garnish with parsley before serving.

NOTE: Length of cooking time depends on type of dish used and size of fillets. Do *not* use foil-lined pan for this recipe as fish and sauce will pick up metallic taste.

4 SERVINGS (1 SERVING = 4 OUNCES)

Stuffed Peppers

DAY 7

Use the same ingredients as for Stuffed Cabbage Rolls (page 333), substituting 4 small green peppers for the cabbage.

1. Preheat the oven to 325° F.

2. Remove the stems, seeds and ribs from the peppers so that they are open shells. Parcook the peppers for 1 minute in boiling water, drain in colander and immediately submerge them in cold water for 10 minutes. Drain peppers upside down on paper towel until ready to use.

3. Prepare the stuffing and carefully stuff each pepper with one-quarter of the meat mixture. Place the peppers in a small casserole, slightly deeper than the height of the peppers.

4. Mix together the tomato sauce mixture and pour over the peppers (Step 6 in the Stuffed Cabbage Rolls recipe).

5. Bake, covered, for 1½ hours. Remove the cover during the last 15 minutes of cooking time. If the sauce has not thickened, then reduce it in a saucepan. Pour over the peppers and serve immediately.

NOTE: This dish benefits in taste if it is cooked 1 day in advance.

4 SERVINGS (1 SERVING = 1 PEPPER)

The Southampton Maintenance Diet Recipes

Strawberry or Banana Yogurt Freeze

DAYS 1 AND 6

1 cup plain low-fat yogurt
1 serving fruit (½ cup fresh or frozen unsweetened
    strawberries, or ½ banana)

1. Mix ingredients in blender.
2. Pour into ice-cube tray and place in freezer 2 to 3 hours, until solid.
3. Allow to soften slightly and puree in blender before eating.

NOTE: If desired, ½ cup fresh or canned (unsweetened) pineapple, in its own juice, with juice drained, may be substituted for the other fruits.

1 SERVING

Yogurt Topping

DAY 2

½ cup yogurt
1½ tablespoons unsweetened apple juice
Pinch of cinnamon
Pinch of freshly grated nutmeg
Yield: 9½ tablespoons

Mix all ingredients thoroughly and chill until ready
for use.

1 SERVING = 1 TABLESPOON

Fruit Shake

DAYS 2–5, 7

1 cup skim milk, or 1 cup plain low-fat yogurt
1 serving fruit (½ banana, or ½ cup fresh or frozen
unsweetened raspberries or blueberries, or ½ cup fresh
or canned unsweetened pineapple, or ½ cup mango)

1. Add 1 cup skim milk or 1 cup plain low-fat yogurt
to 1 serving of fruit.
2. Add 3 ice cubes. Mix in blender until smooth.

1 SERVING

Pineapple Ice

DAY 6

1 cup unsweetened pineapple (canned in its own juice)
Garnish: 2 fresh mint leaves

339

1. Puree pineapple and juice in blender or food processor. Pour into ice-cube trays. Freeze until solid.

2. Remove from freezer, allow to soften slightly. Puree mixture in blender. Serve in glass goblets, garnished with fresh mint leaf.

NOTE: If desired, this recipe can be used with any other suitable fruits served at dinner. For example, with a pear (canned, unsweetened) on Day 1 or a peach (canned, unsweetened) on Day 4.

2 SERVINGS

APPENDIX

Measurement Chart

Standard Weights and Measures

Volume (for liquids)

Dash	= 8 drops
1 tablespoon	= 3 teaspoons
1 fluid ounce	= 2 tablespoons
¼ cup (2 fluid ounces)	= 4 tablespoons
⅓ cup	= 5⅓ tablespoons
½ cup (4 fluid ounces)	= 8 tablespoons
1 cup (8 fluid ounces)	= 16 tablespoons

Weight (for solids)

1 pound	= 16 ounces

NOTE: These are based on level measurements. When measuring liquids, vegetables, fruits, cottage cheese and canned fish use measuring cups (preferably standard U.S. measuring cups, such as Foley). Solids such as fresh meats and fish should be weighed on a scale.

THE ROLE OF VITAMINS

VITAMIN AND MINERAL SUPPLEMENTS are generally recommended during weight reduction. According to the Committee on Dietary Allowances and the Food and Nutrition Board of the National Academy of Sciences (1980 edition of Recommended Dietary Allowances, National Academy of Sciences):

. . . those who, for one reason or another, reduce their calorie consumption below the average energy allowance for their age or sex would need to select foods having a higher nutrient concentration than the RDA/1000 kcal. For example, a 1,000-calorie weight-reduction diet, in order to be nutritionally adequate, would have to supply most nutrients in at least double the allowance per thousand calories, an objective that is difficult to achieve without supplementation.

THE ROLE OF EXERCISE

A WELL-DESIGNED PROGRAM of moderate exercise is recommended for Southampton Dieters. This should consist both of aerobic and body-toning exercise.

The Southampton Diet is essentially a low-fat diet designed to prevent heart and blood vessel diseases. Aerobic exercise is another preventive measure for such diseases that should be considered by every dieter.

Body-toning exercise is of value to those concerned with body definition.

345

THE ROLE OF DRUGS

IF YOU HAVE DIFFICULTY remaining on the Southampton Diet—or losing weight—it may be caused by the ingestion of a drug that stimulates appetite or causes water retention. Any one of the following drugs might produce these effects:

	Generic Name	Brand Name
Antidepressants	amitriptyline	Amitril
		Elavil
		Endep
		Rolavil
	doxepin hydrochloride	Adapin
		Sinequan
	imipramine	Antipress
		Presamine
		Ropamine
		Tofranil
		Triavil
	thioridazine hydrochloride	Mellaril
Antihypertensives	clonidine	Catapres
	guanethidine sulfate	Ismelin
	methyldopa	Aldomet
Anticonvulsants	phenytoin	Dilantin
Antiinflammatory Agents	oxyphenbutazone	Oxalid
		Tandearil
	phenylbutazone	Azolid
		Butazolidin

	Generic Name	Brand Name
Conjugated	estrogen	DES
Hormones		Estrate
		Estrocon
		Femest
		Kestrin
		Menotabs
		Ovest
		Palopause
		Premarin
	progesterone	Provera
	(medroxyprogesterone	
	acetate)	

All *oral contraceptives* cause changes in weight due to retention of water.

Nonsteroid	fenoprofer calcium	Nalfon
Antiinflammatory	ibuprofen	Motrin
Agents	naproxen	Naprosyn
	tolmetin sodium	Tolectin
Steroids	methylprednisolone	Medrol
	prednisone	Deltasone
		Lisacort
		Meticorten
		Paracort
		Sterapred
Sedatives	flurazepam	Dalmane
Tranquilizers	chlordiazepoxide	Chlordia zachel
		Librium
		Tenax
	clorazepate	Azene
		Tranxene
	diazepam	Valium
	oxazepam	Serax

SPECIAL ILLNESSES REQUIRING SPECIAL DIETS

THE DIETARY REQUIREMENTS of those who are afflicted with the following diseases have *not* been provided for on the Southampton Diet program. An individualized physician-designed diet should be made available for anyone who suffers from:

Hypertension
Congestive heart failure
Atherosclerotic vessel disease
Congenital or genetic diseases of excess fat or lipids
Diabetes mellitus, thyroid disease and other endocrine disorders
Diverticulosis
Diverticulitis
Emphysema
Gallbladder disease
Renal disease
Food allergies

These are the most common diseases for which special diets should be prescribed.

INDEX

INDEX

acetyl choline, dopamine blocked by, 74
activities list, as behavior technique, 96–97
adolescence, dieting in, 233
aggressive behavior, 66
alcohol, 18, 110, 130
  as sad food, 76
  see also wine
amino acids, 38, 41, 42–43, 62–76, 110, 224, 234
  chemical formula for, 63
  defined, 63
  essential, 64
  fluctuation in blood levels of, 67
  molecular structure of, 63
  nonessential, 64
  nutritional importance of, 64
  R factor in, 63
  tryptophan, 65–66, 67, 70, 72–73, 75, 224, 228, 233
  tyrosine, 71, 75, 76
  see also neurotransmitters
amphetamines, 24, 33
anger, 59
  overeating as response to, 18, 19–21, 34–35
anticonvulsants, 346
antidepressants, 61, 66, 346
antihypertensives, 346

antiinflammatory agents, 346
antipasto salad, 261–62
anxiety, 35, 96–97, 110
  caffeine and, 112, 225
  Fat Shield against, 27, 36, 47–48
appearance:
  beauty standards and, 11, 84
  falling in love and, 77
  sexual desirability and, 83–84
  studies of perceptions of, 55
  success and, 12, 14, 15, 55, 84
appetite:
  depression as factor in, 28, 37, 38, 53–54, 61
  happiness as factor in, 77
  true hunger vs., 41
apples, baked, 329
applesauce, unsweetened, 332–33
artichoke salad, 268–69
asparagus:
  chicken and, with mustard dressing, 280
  cold, with Roquefort, 254–55
  stir-fry chicken with, 295–96
avocados, ripe, as sad food, 76

Bacall, Lauren, 13
baking, baked, 110, 129, 230, 239
  apple, 329
  chicken breast, 242–43

baking, baked (*cont.*)
  chicken with lemon and herbs,
    303–4
  fish, 241
  fish with mushrooms in a
    package, 288–89
  fish with tomato sauce, 336–37
  lamb shanks with new potatoes,
    307
  salmon mousse, 250
bananas, 111
  as happy food, 75
  yogurt freeze, 338
bass:
  poached, 270–71
  steamed, 291–92
beans:
  fermented black, 172
  see also string beans
beansprouts, 171
  chicken and, with sesame
    dressing, 284
Beard, James, 13
beauty, changing standards of,
  11, 84
beef:
  aged, as sad food, 76
  as happy food, 75, 225
  stir-fry, with broccoli, 298–99
  stock, 113
beer, as sad food, 76
beets, 239
  cold pickled, 332
  soup, 334
behavioral techniques, 25, 29, 43–
  45, 90–102, 226
  activities list as, 96–97
  confrontation method as, 97–98
  food diary as, 100–101
  for food preparation, 93–94
  for high visual sensitivity, 94–95
  punishments and rewards as,
    99–100
  replacement method as, 96–97,
    98

  for situational stimuli, 95–96
  time-stretch method as, 98–99
  use of mirror and, 101
"Being Good to Yourself"
  program, 59
Berger, Stuart:
  family background of, 16–20,
    48
  weight problem of, 12, 14, 15–
    26, 36, 48, 56, 68–69, 92,
    98
Berscheid, Ellen, 55
blood pressure, 32
bluefish, grilled, 266–67
boiling, 239
bok choy (Chinese cabbage), 171
boredom, overeating and, 96–97
borscht, 334
bouillabaisse, 259–60
bouillon, instant, 228
bouquet garni, 249
brain:
  biochemistry of, 24, 25, 41, 61–
    76; *see also* amino acids;
    neurotransmitters
  ketones and, 32
braised leeks, 255–56
bran cereals, 111, 226
bread, 129, 224, 225–26
  butter on, 207
  whole-grain, 111, 226
breakfasts, 224
  choice of, 110, 114, 142
  in Maintenance Diet, 207, 208
breast feeding, 78, 233
Brin, Myron, 68*n*
broccoli, 239
  chicken and, with mustard
    dressing, 280
  as happy food, 71, 75
  salad, 265
  stir-fry, 292
  stir-fry chicken or beef with,
    298–99
  vinaigrette, 252–53

broiling, broiled, 110, 113, 129,
    230
  chicken breast, 240
  fish, 242
  turkey or veal, 264–65
broth, noodles with, 286
brown rice:
  as happy food, 71, 75
  recipe for, 238
brussels sprouts, as happy food,
    75
buckwheat groats (kasha), 328
butter, 130, 144, 207, 230, 232
buttermilk, 113
B vitamins:
  absorption of, 234
  deficiencies of, 67–68, 73
  sources of, 71–72, 75

cabbage:
  Chinese, 171–72
  stuffed, 333–34
caffeine, in beverages, 112,
    225
calorie counters, 23, 27
calories, 23–24, 25
  orgasm and, 81
  snacks and, 73
candies, dietetic, 226
canned food:
  fresh vs., 111
  labels on, 112
  packing liquid for, 111–12, 231
cantaloupe, as happy food, 75
cappuccino, 152, 263
carbohydrates, 110, 224, 233, 234
  diets high in, 67
  diets low in, 32–33
  tryptophan and, 67, 70, 224
career problems, overweight and,
    42, 52–55
carrots, 239
  simmered, 279
  stir-fry, 292
catsup, 113

cauliflower, 239
  puree, 247
cereals, 226
  bran, 111, 226
chayote, 189–90
  steamed, with tomato sauce,
    320
cheese:
  aged, as sad food, 76
  cottage, 70, 111, 113, 224, 225
  cream, 231
  croque-monsieur (melted
    cheese sandwich), 252
  crostini (toasted cheese
    sandwich), 268
  fruit and, 259
  grilled feta sandwich, 303
  as happy food, 71, 75
  Monterey Jack, 189, 315, 321
  Muenster, 189
  sandwiches, 252, 268, 303
  sliced tomatoes and, with basil,
    273
chewing, 98, 232
chewing gum, 226–27
Chianti, as sad food, 76
chicken, 110, 237
  and asparagus (or broccoli)
    salad with mustard dressing,
    280
  baked, with lemon and herbs,
    303–4
  baked breast of, 242–43
  with bean sprout salad with
    sesame dressing, 284
  breasts picante con chiles (spicy
    with chiles), 317
  breasts tarragon, poached, 246
  broiled breast of, 240
  and cucumber salad with
    sesame dressing, 284
  enchiladas, 323
  Greek-style, 314
  grilled, 269
  as happy food, 70, 75

chicken (*cont.*)
lime, 321–22
liver, chopped, 336
poached, 237, 246
in a pot, 335
salad, 305
skin removed from, 112, 129, 228
steamed, 294–95
stir-fry, with asparagus, 295–96
stir-fry, with broccoli, 298–99
stock, 113, 161–62, 227
tacos, 315
teriyaki, 277–78
yakitori with vegetables, 282–83
chick-peas, as sad food, 74, 76
children:
eating patterns of, 16–21, 47–48
unattractive, 55
chiles (chili pepper), 189, 190
chicken breasts picante con, 317
chilled cucumber-yogurt soup, 313
Chinese menu, 171–80
recipes for, 290–99
Chinese vegetable salad, 293–94
chocolate:
as sad food, 25, 39–40, 69, 73, 76
as substitute for emotional needs, 73, 78–79
cholesterol, 224–25
choline:
drawbacks of, 73–74
sources of, 74, 76
chopped chicken liver, 336
chopsticks, 171
as time-stretch technique, 98
Claiborne, Craig, 13
clam soup, 272–73
club soda, 110, 130, 231
codfish steaks in tomato sauce, 274
coffee, 112

decaffeinated, 110, 112, 113, 152, 225
iced, 113
Italian, 152, 263
coleslaw salad, 327
constipation, 230
contract, Southampton Diet, 103–5
contractual dieting, 100
cooked (poached) chicken or turkey breasts for sandwiches, salads or snacks, 237
cooking tips, 110, 112–13
for ethnic menus, 143–44, 161–163, 173, 190
cottage cheese, 111, 113
as happy food, 70, 224
selection of, 225
crab:
canned, 112
three-flavor vinegar, 276
cranberry-fruit relish, 326
cream:
sour, 76, 232
sweet, 232
cream cheese, 231
croque-monsieur (melted cheese sandwich), 252
crostini (toasted cheese sandwich), 268
cucumbers:
chicken and, with sesame dressing, 284
and radishes with sesame dressing, 282
salad, 329
salad, spicy, 295
sauce, 257
and yogurt salad, 306
yogurt soup, chilled, 313

dancers, weight problem of, 52–55
dashi, 161–62

death:
  fad diets and, 32
  obesity and, 11–12
dehydration, 32
depression:
  biochemical components of,
    24, 25, 39–40; see also amino
    acids; neurotransmitters; sad
    foods
  characteristics of, 50, 53–54
  dieting and, 28, 38, 69
  increased appetite due to, 28,
    37, 38, 53–54, 61
  overweight as cause of, 48–49,
    53, 55, 59, 71, 83
  postpartum, 39
  sleep patterns and, 66
  studies of, 65–66, 68
  vitamin deficiencies and, 67–68
deprivation:
  diet as, 31, 37
  overeating as response to, 18,
    19–21, 31, 37, 48
desserts, 130
  baked apple, 329
  pineapple ice, 339–40
  poached pears in wine, 254
  timing of, 72
diaries, food, 100–101
diet pills, 33, 227–28
  amphetamines as, 24, 33
diets:
  in adolescence, 233
  biochemical factors in, 15, 24–
    25, 26, 28–29, 39–43, 61–76
  discipline and, 28, 56,
  fad, 15, 23, 27, 31–33, 37, 38,
    39, 49
  failure of, 18, 30, 32–33, 38, 42,
    43, 49
  five fundamentals of, 102
  group method of, 41–42
  high carbohydrate, 67
  high protein, 32–33
  low carbohydrate, 32–33

  low protein, 67
  medical disorders and, 233, 348
  missing link in, 62–63
  nutritional factors in, 15, 23–
    24, 26, 31–35, 64, 68, 233
  pregnancy and, 233
  psychological factors in, 15, 24–
    25, 26, 27–28, 35–40, 46–60
  vegetarian, 68
  yo-yo problem and, 25, 32–33,
    48, 56, 57
diet sodas, 112, 226
diuretics, 227–28
divorce, 55
dizziness, 32, 74
dolmitas (stuffed grape leaves),
    312–13
dopamine, 66, 68, 71
dressings, see salad dressings
drowsiness, 73, 74
drugs, 18, 346–47
  antidepressants, 61, 66, 347
  diet pills, 24, 33, 7–28
  neurochemical research and,
    61
  sleeping pills, 66, 347

eating patterns, 226
  childhood, 16–21, 47–48
  ethnic influences on, 18–20,
    51–52
  food as self-punishment and,
    19–21
  gobbling as, 44, 98
  stimulas/response dynamic in,
    91–98
eggplant:
  salad, 302
  stuffed, 309–10
eggs, as happy foods, 71, 72, 75
enchiladas, 190
  chicken, 323
energy:
  dieting and, 14, 25, 37
  thinness and, 12

ensalada (salad), 316–17, 318–19
  with tuna or turkey, 319
espresso, 152
Ethnic Diets, 111, 139–205, 207,
  228
  recipes for, 244–337
ethnic homes, emphasis on food
  in 18–20, 51–52
Euphoria Plateau, 56–58
exercise, 233, 345
  sex as, 81–83

family, weight problems and, 16–
  20, 34–35, 51–52
fasting, disadvantages of, 231
fatigue:
  dieting and, 28, 32, 37, 63, 68
  mineral deficiencies and, 72
  vitamin deficiencies and, 68
fats, 112, 224–25, 228, 232
  cooking without, 110, 113, 130,
    144
  in Maintenance Diet, 207,
    230
  as sad foods, 73–74
  seasoning pans with, 232
  see also butter; margarine; oil
Fat Shield, 27–28, 35–40, 46–60,
  91
  anxiety and, 27, 36, 47–48
  career problems and, 52–55
  defined, 27, 35–36, 47
  intimacy and, 47, 48, 55, 59
  sex and, 36, 47, 59, 77–78,
    83
fiber, 111, 228, 232
fish, 110, 112, 144, 224–25
  baked, 241
  baked, with mushrooms in a
    package, 288–89
  baked, with tomato sauce, 336–
    337
  baked salmon mousse, 250
  bouillabaisse, 259–60
  broiled, 242
  canned, 111–12, 231
  codfish steaks in tomato sauce,
    274
  defrosting of, 161
  gefilte, 330
  grilled bluefish, 266–67
  as happy food, 71, 72, 75
  plaki, 310–11
  sake simmered, 281
  spigola bollito (poached bass),
    270–71
  steamed fillet of sole with
    fennel, 253
  steamed sea bass or red
    snapper, 291–92
  stew, 259–60, 305–6
  stock, 113
  teriyaki, 288
  tuna salad, 266
folic acid:
  sources of, 71, 75
  vitamin C combined with, 68,
    71
food preparation:
  behavioral techniques for, 93–
    94
  cooking techniques and, 110,
    112–13, 143–44, 162–63, 173,
    230, 237, 238–39
  presentation and, 144, 161
food processors, 144
four-point program, 23, 26–76
  behavioral techniques in, 29,
    43–45, 90–102
  diet itself in 26, 31–35, 91
  Fat Shield in, 27–28, 35–40,
    46–60, 91
  mood/food link in, 28–29, 40–
    43, 61–76, 91
  summary of, 26–29
Franey, Pierre, 13
freezes, 233, 234
  strawberry or banana yogurt,
    338
French and nouvelle cuisine
    menu, 143–51
  recipes for, 244–60

fruit juice:
  as substitute for fruit, 110,
    232
  unsweetened, 110, 111, 229
fruits, 71, 75, 130
  canned, 111, 130, 229
  dried, 231
  fresh vs. processed, 111
  et fromage (with cheese), 259
  frozen, 111, 229
  as happy foods, 71, 75
  salad, 273, 308
  shake, 339
  substitutes for, 110, 232
  in yogurt, 233
  see also specific kinds of fruit
frustration, 59
  overeating as response to, 18,
    19–21
frying, 230
  see also stir-fry

gamma aminobutyric acid
    (GABA), 74, 76
garlic, selection of, 153
garnishes, 162
gefilte fish, 330
Gelenberg, Alan J., 66n
ginger, fresh, 172
ginger juice, 162
glucose, 32, 72, 110, 224
  MSG and, 74
  physical effects of, 39–40
  see also sugar
gobbling, 44, 98
Good Cook series, 239
grains:
  as happy foods, 71, 72, 75
  kasha, 328
  see also cereals; rice
grapefruit, as happy food, 75
grape leaves, stuffed, 312–13
gratin aux zucchini (zucchini
    with cheese), 260
gravies, 129, 230

Greek menu, 181–88
  recipes for, 300–14
green beans, see string beans
grilled food:
  bluefish, 266–67
  chicken, 268
  feta sandwich, 303
  tomatoes with rosemary, 251–
    252
Growdon, John H., 65n
Guerard, Michel, 143
gum, chewing, 226–27

happiness, 55, 56
  appetite decreased by, 77
  thinness and, 12, 14–15
happy foods, 25, 28, 41, 69, 70–
    72, 224, 225
  list of, 75
  in Maintenance Diet, 207
Harvard School of Public Health,
    24, 31
Harvard University, depression
    studies at, 66
headaches, 74
health:
  caring for yourself and, 59, 84
  fad diets as danger to, 23, 27,
    31–33, 49
  fasting and, 231
  obesity and, 11–12
heart, as happy food, 71, 75
heart disease, 12
helplessness, attempts at weight
    loss and, 36–37, 38, 39–40,
    49, 50
herbs and spices, 112–13, 130, 239
herb tea, 110, 113, 225, 229
herring, pickled, as sad food, 76
homeostasis, 31
hormones, conjugated, 347
hunger, 226
  appetite vs., 41
  stimuli of food vs., 91–92
hypoglycemia, 72

ice, pineapple, 339–40
illnesses, special diets for, 233,
    348
infants, sensual stimulation of, 78
insomnia, serotonin and, 66
insulin:
    defined, 72
    tryptophan levels and, 72–73
intimacy:
    Fat Shield as barrier against,
        47, 48, 55, 59
    food as substitute for, 78–79
iron deficiency, 72
irritability, 42
    low blood sugar and, 72
    sleeping pills and, 66
isoleucine, 73
Italian dressing, 262
Italian menu, 152–60
    recipes for, 261–75

Japanese menu, 161–70
    recipes for, 276–89
Jewish menu, 198–205
    recipes for, 326–37

kasha, 328
ketones, 32
ketonic diet, 32–33
ketosis, 32
kidney, as happy food, 71, 75
kidney damage, 32

lactobacillus culture, 234
lamb, 225
    baked shanks with new
        potatoes, 307
Lauren, Ralph, 13
lecithin, drawbacks of, 73–74
leeks, braised, 255–56
lemon juice, 239
    as basting ingredient, 113
    as salad dressing, 112, 130, 229
lemons, 225
    as happy food, 75

lentils, as sad food, 74, 76
lethargy, 42
    GABA as cause of, 74
    increased appetite due to, 37
    vitamin deficiencies and, 68
leucine, 73
lime(s):
    chicken 321–22
    as happy food, 75
liquid vs. solid measurements, 228
liver:
    chopped chicken, as happy
        food, 71, 75
    sugar storage in, 74
lobster, as sad food, 74, 76
loneliness, 17–18, 55–56, 59, 86–
    87
love, 59, 89
    chocolate as substitute for, 73
    falling in, 77, 78–79

magnesium, 72
margarine, 130, 207, 232
    diet, 232
marital problems, weight gains
    and, 55, 79–83
masturbation, 85–86
mayonnaise, 232
    diet, 232
    as sad food, 74
meals:
    preparation of, 93–94
    proper environment for, 95–96
    skipping of, 110, 224
    switching of, 224, 230, 234
    timing of, 72, 110, 224, 229,
        230–31, 234
measuring cups, 111, 228, 231–32
meats:
    cooking techniques for, 230
    as happy food, 71, 72, 75
    lean cuts of, 112, 113, 129
    marbled, as sad food, 73, 74, 76
    organ, 71, 72, 75

red, 71, 75
see also beef; lamb; veal
Mediterranean fish stew, 305–6
memory, vitamin B$_{12}$ and, 68
Mexican menu, 189–97
  recipes for, 315–25
Mexican rice, 318
milk:
  buttermilk, 113
  as happy food, 25, 69, 71, 72,
    75
  in Maintenance Diet, 207
  skim, 111, 112, 207, 225, 226
minerals, 345–46
mineral water, 130, 152–53
  as substitute, 110
mirrors, behavioral techniques
  and, 101
MIT, amino acid studies by, 65–
  66, 67
monosodium glutamate (MSG),
  74, 76, 112
Monterey Jack cheese, 189, 315,
  321
mood:
  biochemical factors in, 24–25,
    28–29, 37–43, 61–76, 91, 224,
    231
  after fad dieting, 38
moules à la marinière (mussels
  in wine), 258
mussels:
  soup, 272–73
  in wine, 258
mustard dressing, 280

neurochemistry:
  mood and, 24, 61–76
  revolutionary impact of, 61–62
neurotransmitters, 64–69
  defined, 64
  dopamine as, 66, 68, 71
  functioning of, 64–65
  GABA as, 74, 76
  norepinephrine as, 66

phenylalanine as, 73, 76, 78
positive vs. negative, 64–65
serotonin, 65–66, 67, 71
New York University, 25, 31
niacin (vitamin B$_3$), sources of,
  71
niçoise salad, 244–45
nonsteroid antiinflammatory
  agents, 348
noodles:
  with broth, 287
  transparent, 172
norepinephrine, 66
nouvelle cuisine menu, 143–51
  recipes for, 244–60

obesity:
  author's experience with, 12,
    14, 15–26, 36, 48, 56, 68–69,
    92, 98
  coital positions and, 87–88
  emotional problems as cause
    of, 17–21, 27–28, 34–35, 36–
    37, 46–48
  emotional stress due to, 19, 21–
    22, 36, 47, 48, 49–55
  incidence of, 30
  as intractable medical problem,
    24, 90
  misperceptions of, 36
  mortality rate and, 11–12
  in parents, 18
  self-delusions and, 22
  sense of helplessness and, 36–
    37, 38, 49, 50
oil, 130, 144, 207
  in salad dressings, 112, 207, 230
O'Keeffe, Georgia, 13
Onassis, Jacqueline Kennedy, 13
onion soup, 256
oral contraceptives, 348
oral gratification, 20, 22, 47–48,
  53, 78
orgasms, 81, 84
oysters, as happy food, 71

pans, nonstick, 113, 144, 173, 227,
     230, 239
  seasoning of, 232
Parkinson's disease, 66
parties, dieting at, 44, 231
pasta, buying of, 152
pâté, veal, 248
Pavlov, Ivan Petrovich, 91
pears, poached, in wine, 254
Peking salad, 290–91
peppers:
  chili, 189, 190
  green, 71, 75
  as happy food, 71, 75
  roasted red, in salad, 271–72
  stuffed, 337
pineapple, 111
  as happy food, 75
  ice, 339–40
pizza Southampton, 264
poaching, poached, 110, 129, 144,
     230
  bass, 270–71
  chicken breasts tarragon,
     246
  chicken or turkey breasts for
     sandwiches, salads or snacks,
     237
  pears in wine, 254
Pollock, Jackson, 13
pompano en salsa verde (in green
     tomato sauce), 324–25
pork, 75
potassium, 49, 72
potatoes, 239
  baked lamb shanks with, 307
  topping for, 113
pots, types of, 238–39
poultry:
  as happy food, 70, 72, 75
  skin of, 112, 129, 228
  white meat vs. dark meat of,
     112
  see also chicken; turkey
pregnancy, dieting and, 232

protein:
  amino acids as building blocks
     of, 63, 67
  diets low in, 67
  impairment of production of,
     32, 64
  ketosis and, 32
  liquid, 33
prune juice, 231
psychosomatic medicine, 58
psychotherapy, weight loss and,
     25, 46, 54, 90
punishment:
  as behavioral technique, 99
  overeating as response to, 19–
     20
  self-, 15, 19–21, 22, 28, 35, 38,
     47, 48–49, 59, 79; see also Fat
     Shield
puree, pureed, 144
  cauliflower, 247
  tomato sauce, 251

quesadillas, 190, 321

Radziwill, Lee, 13
ratatouille, 249
red snapper:
  steamed, 291–92
  Veracruz, 323–24
reinforcement, positive, 100
relish, cranberry-fruit, 326
replacement method, as
     behavioral technique, 96–97,
     98
restaurants:
  eating in, see Southampton
     Restaurant and Vacation
     Menu
  in Hamptons, 13
reward(s):
  as behavioral technique, 99–
     100
  food as, 18–19, 51

riboflavin (vitamin B$_2$):
  deficiency of, 68
  sources of, 71–72
rice, 110, 161
  brown, 71, 75, 238
  crackers and cakes, 162, 172
  as happy food, 71, 75
  Mexican, 318
  saffron, 302
  white, 278
  wild, 243
rice bran, as happy food, 71, 75
roasted red pepper salad, 271–72
Rubens, Peter Paul, 11

sad foods, 25, 28, 39–40, 41, 69,
    70, 72–74
  list of, 76
saffron rice, 302
sake, 162
  simmered fish, 281
salad dressings, 112, 130, 229, 230
  chili, 316–17
  commercial, 112, 229–30
  Greek, 300–301
  Italian, 262
  lemon juice as, 112, 130, 229
  mustard, 280
  oil in, 112, 207, 230
  Peking, 290–91
  sesame, 282, 284
  vinaigrette, 245
salads, 110, 237
  antipasto, 261–62
  artichoke, 268–69
  broccoli, 265
  chicken, 305
  chicken and asparagus (or
    broccoli), with mustard
    dressing, 280
  chicken and beansprout with
    sesame dressing, 284
  Chinese vegetable, 293–94
  coleslaw, 327
  cucumber, 329

  cucumber and yogurt, 306
  cucumbers and radishes with
    sesame dressing, 282
  eggplant, 302
  fruit, 273, 308
  Greek, 300–301
  Greek fruit, 308
  green brean, 265
  green bean with sesame
    dressing, 282
  Mexican, 316–17, 318–19
  mixed green, 110, 152, 226
  niçoise, 244–45
  Peking, 290–91
  roasted red pepper, 271–72
  shrimp and tomato, 308
  sliced tomato, with basil and
    oregano, 267
  sliced tomatoes and mozzarella
    cheese with basil, 273
  sliced tomatoes with cucumber
    sauce, 257
  spicy cucumber, 295
  spinach with sesame dressing,
    282
  tofu, 286
  tuna, 266, 305
salmon:
  canned, 112
  as happy food, 71
  mousse, baked, 250
salsa, 190, 315–16, 322
salsa verde, 324–25
salt, 112, 130, 153, 162, 229
sandwiches, 237
  cheese, 252, 268, 303
  croque-monsieur (melted
    cheese), 252
  crostini (toasted cheese), 268
  grilled feta, 303
sauces, 129, 143, 144, 230
  cucumber, 257
  salsa, 190, 315–16, 322
  salsa verde (green tomato
    sauce), 324–25

sauces (*cont.*)
  teriyaki, 277
  tomato, light, 262–63
  tomato, pureed, 251
  yakitori, 283
sautéeing, sautéed, 113, 239
  snow peas with shallots and
    basil, 247–48
scales, for weighing food, 111,
  228
scallops:
  stir-fry, with mushrooms and
    red pepper, 297–98
  yakitori with vegetables, 285
sedatives, 347
seesaw problem, *see* yo-yo
  problem
self-destructive behavior,
  overeating as, 18, 19–21, 28,
  35, 37
senses, sexuality and, 84–85
serotonin, 65–66, 67
  replenishment of, 66, 71
sesame dressing, 282, 284
sesame seeds, toasting of, 162–63
sex, 77–89
  afterplay and, 88–89
  chocolate as substitute for, 73
  eating compared to, 78
  as exercise, 81–83
  Fat Shield, against, 36, 47, 59,
    77–78, 83
  foreplay and, 88
  initiating encounters and, 86
  positions for obese in, 87–88
  satisfying encounters and, 78,
    84–85, 88–89
  self-exploration and, 85–86
  social life and, 86
sexual revolution, social effects
  of, 87
shakes, 233, 234
  fruit, 339
shopping tips, 111–12
  for ethnic menus, 143–44, 153,
161–63, 171–72, 181, 189–90,
  198
shrimp:
  canned, 112
  marinara, 262
  Mykonos, 301
  stir-fry, with snow peas, 296–97
  three-flavor vinegar, 276
  and tomato salad, 308
shyness, 17–18
Silverstone cookware, 227
simmered string beans or carrots,
  279
situational stimuli, food
  consumption and, 95–96
skewers, disposable bamboo, 162
Skinner, B. F., 91
sleep, tryptophan and, 66
sleeping pills, 66, 347
sliced tomatoes:
  with cucumber sauce, 256
  and mozzarella cheese with
    basil, 273
  salad with basil and oregano,
    267
snacks:
  afternoon, 114, 142, 209
  energy expenditure and, 73
  evening, 110, 114, 142, 209
  in Maintenance Diet, 207, 209
  moods and, 25
  morning, 209
  response to situational stimuli
    and, 95
  sex and, 88–89
  skipping of, 110
  sugar blues and, 72
  time-stretch techniques and, 99
  timing of, 110, 224, 229, 234
snow peas, 171
  sautéed, with shallots and
    basil, 247–48
  stir-fry shrimp with, 296–97
soda:
  Bitter Lemon, 231

club, 110, 130, 231
diet, 112, 226
tonic water, 231
sodium, water retention and, 32–
33, 229
sole, steamed fillet of, with
fennel, 253
solid vs. liquid measurement, 228
soup, 129
beet, 334
chilled cucumber-yogurt, 313
clam, 272–73
mussel, 272–73
onion, 256
vermicelli, 293
see also stew; stock
sour cream, 232
as sad food, 76
Southampton, N.Y.:
as chic resort area, 12–14
dieters' demands in, 14
stresses on residents of, 48
Southampton Diet:
birth of, 11–29
caring for yourself as basis of,
59, 84
contract for, 42, 103–5
Ethnic, 111, 139–205, 207, 228,
244–337
Euphoria Plateau and, 56–58
as four-point program, see four-
point program
how to stay on, 90–102
menus for, 115–28
primitive version of, 25
questions and answers for, 224–
234
recipes for, 237–337
snacks and, 72, 73, 95, 110, 114,
229
as stress-free, 27, 42–43, 62–76,
110
substitute items and, 110, 111
success of, 26, 27, 29, 30–45
as turning point, 103–4

uniqueness of, 37, 41, 61, 62,
64
unlimited items on, 109
Week 1 of, 110, 113–21, 228
Week 2 of, 111, 113–14, 122–
28, 141, 228
weight loss of four to ten
pounds and, 16, 26, 44
weight loss of more than ten
pounds and, 26, 27, 29, 35,
43, 49–52, 56–58
Southampton Maintenance Diet,
111, 113, 206–23, 233
breakfasts and snacks for, 207,
208–9
for men, 217–23
questions and answers for, 230,
232
recipes for, 338–40
two plans of, 207
for women, 210–16
Southampton Restaurant and
Vacation Menu, 110, 129–37
guidelines for, 129–30
questions and answers for, 229,
230
substitute items and, 130
soybeans:
noodles made from, 172
soy sauce, 161, 162, 172
spices, see herbs and spices
spicy cucumber salad, 295
spigola bollito (poached bass),
270–71
spinach:
garlic-flavored, 274–75
as happy food, 75
with sesame dressing, 282
steamed, with dill and lemon,
304
sprays, nonstick 227
spritzers, 110, 130, 227
squash, 239
chayote, 189–90, 320
starvation, 23, 32

steaming, steamed, 129
  chicken, 294–95
  fillet of sole with fennel, 253
  fresh vegetables, 238–39
  red snapper, 291–92
  sea bass, 291–92
  spinach, sliced raw tomatoes or
    steamed zucchini with dill
    and lemon, 304
  zucchini or chayote with
    tomato sauce, 320
steroids, 347
stew:
  fish, 259–60
  Mediterranean fish, 305–6
stir-fry:
  beef with broccoli, 298–99
  broccoli, carrots or string
    beans, 292
  chicken with asparagus, 295–96
  chicken with broccoli, 298–99
  scallops with mushrooms and
    red pepper, 297–98
  shrimp with snow peas, 296–97
stock, 144, 227
  as basting ingredient, 113
  dashi as, 161–62
stomach stapling, 24, 34
strawberries:
  freeze, 338
  as happy food, 71, 75
string beans:
  salad, 265
  with sesame dressing, 282
  simmered, 279
  stir-fry, 292
stuffed foods:
  cabbage rolls, 333–34
  eggplant, 309–10
  grape leaves, 312–13
  peppers, 337
  rib veal chops, 327–28
sublimation, 20–21, 78
success, physical appearance and,
  12, 14, 15, 55, 84

sugar, 110, 224, 231
  blues, 39–40, 72–73, 76
  MSG and, 74
  in processed foods, 111, 112,
    113, 160, 226, 229
  vitamin depletion and, 72
  see also glucose
suicide rate, 12
surgical procedures for obesity,
  24, 34
sweeteners, artificial, 112, 225

tacos, 190
  turkey, chicken or Monterey
    Jack cheese, 315
Taylor, Elizabeth, 33
tea, 112
  herb, 110, 113, 225, 229
  iced, 113
teriyaki sauce, 277
thiamine (vitamin B$_1$), 68, 71–72
thinness:
  advantages of, 12, 14–15, 84
  eating patterns and, 91–92
  as rational goal, 12, 15
  true hunger and, 41
three-flavor vinegar crab or
  shrimp, 276
thyroid gland, inhibition of, 74,
  76
thyroid pills, 32, 227–28
time-stretch method, as
  behavioral technique, 98–99
tofu salad, 286
tomatoes, 152
  grilled, with rosemary, 251–52
  as happy food, 71
  salad with basil and oregano,
    267
  sliced, and mozzarella cheese
    with basil, 273
  sliced, with cucumber sauce,
    257
  sliced raw, with dill and lemon,
    304

tomato juice:
    as basting ingredient, 113
    as substitute, 110
tomato sauce:
    baked fish with 336–37
    green, 324–25
    light, 262–63
    pureed, 251
tonic water, 231
tonno, 266
tortillas, 189
    fillings for, 190
tranquilizers, 347
tryptophan, 65–66, 67
    insulin's effects on, 72–73
    pills, 228
    sources of, 70, 75, 224, 233
Tufts Medical School, 31
tuna:
    ensalada (salad) with, 319
    salad, 266, 305, 319
    water-packed, 111–12, 231
turkey, 111, 112, 225
    cooking techniques for, 110
    cutlets with cranberry-fruit
        relish, 326
    ensalada (salad) with, 319
    garlic broiled, 264–65
    as happy food, 70, 75
    loaf, 331
    and Monterey Jack cheese
        quesadilla, 321
    poached, 237
    tacos, 315
tyramine, sources of, 76
tyrosine, 76
    sources of, 71, 75

unsweetened applesauce, 332–33

vacations:
    eating during, see Southampton
        Restaurant and Vacation
        Menu
    weight gain during, 44–45, 54

veal, 225
    burger, 270
    chops, stuffed, 327–28
    chops Veracruz, 319–20
    chops vs. breast, 112
    cutlets, 255
    en salsa (in sauce), 322
    garlic broiled, 264–65
    kebabs, 310
    pâté, 248
    stock, 113
veau (veal) à la provençale, 255
vegetables:
    chicken yakitori with, 282–83
    cooking techniques for, 144,
        230, 238–39
    fresh vs. processed, 111, 228
    as happy foods, 71–72, 75
    measuring of, 111
    pureeing of, 144, 247
    ratatouille, 249
    scallops yakitori with, 285
    seasoning of, 207, 239
    steamed fresh, 238–39
    stock from 113, 227
    substitutes for, 110
    see also specific vegetables
Vegetables (Time-Life), 239
vegetarian diets, vitamin
    deficiencies and, 68
V-8 juice, as substitute, 110
vermicelli soup, 293
vinegar, 112, 130
    rice, 162
    wine, 229
vitamin B₁ (thiamine):
    deficiency of, 68
    sources of, 71–72
vitamin B₂ (riboflavin):
    deficiency of, 68
    sources of, 71–72
vitamin B₃ (niacin), sources of,
    71
vitamin B₆, sources of, 71
vitamin B₁₂, sources of, 71

vitamin C:
    folic acid combined with, 68, 71
    sources of, 71, 75
vitamins:
    absorption of, 234
    role of, 345
    sugar's effects on, 73
vomiting, 34

water, 130, 227
    time-stretch technique and, 98–99
water pills, 227–28
water weight, 32–33, 227, 229
Watson, J. B., 91
weighing yourself, 228, 232
weights and measures, 111, 227, 228, 231–32, 343
wheat germ, as happy food, 71, 75
white rice, 278
whole wheat bread, 111, 226
wild rice, 243
wine, 152–53, 231
    Chianti, 76
    cooking, 153
    in Maintenance Diet, 207

sake, 162
vinegar, 229
    white, 110, 130, 153, 227
woks, 173
Wurtman, R. J. and J. J., 65n

yakitori sauce, 283
yeast, as happy food, 71, 75
yogurt, 111, 113, 181
    fruit in, 233
    as happy food, 25, 75, 224
    importance of, 224, 233–34
    topping, 339
yo-yo problem, 25, 32–33, 48, 56, 57

zucchini, 239
    gratin aux (with chesse), 260
    steamed, with dill and lemon, 304
    steamed, with tomato sauce, 320
zuppa di vongole or di cozze (clam or mussel soup), 272–273